How to Prepare
For Old Age

(Without Taking the Fun out of Life)

By

Bernard S. Otis

How To Prepare For Old Age

(Without Taking the Fun out of Life)

For more information, to inquire about rights to this or other works, or to purchase copies for special educational, business, or sales promotional uses please write to:

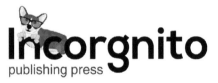

Incorgnito Publishing Press
A division of Market Management Group, LLC
33 S. Wilson Avenue, Suite 113
Pasadena, California 91106
mconant@incorgnitobooks.com

FIRST EDITION

Printed in the United States of America

ISBN: 978-0-9861953-6-5

10 9 8 7 6 5 4 3 2 1

Dedication

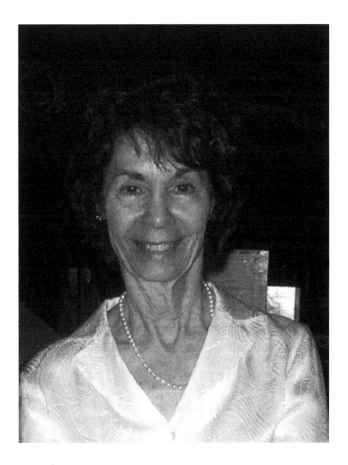

Anna Patricia Otis

April 3, 1941-October 8, 2012

On October 8, 2012, this person, my partner and wife of over 30 years, who was most responsible for whatever accomplishments I have achieved in my life, lost her battle with cancer.

There are not enough words in the dictionary to describe how much she meant to me or the love affair we had from the moment we met in 1983.

Anna was kind, gentle, caring, understanding, and supportive of my efforts to raise myself to highest levels of achievement. Her influence on me cannot be adequately expressed.

She was an internationally recognized teacher of the Senior Visually Impaired and Blind, and she was adored by family, friends, associates, and all who knew her or in some way were touched by her.

None of the successes I have enjoyed since we met would have happened if it had not been for the role she played in my life.

She loved me. There is no way that could've been an easy gig!

Nonetheless, her memory will live on in my mind and heart always, and...

And...

Wait a minute. Wait *one* minute.

I'm going to indulge here.

I'm going to indulge in this dedication a bit further. Why? Because Anna was my beloved wife. She is the sole reason I've written this book, and a pithy few sentences is simply not going to do justice for either her or our close to thirty years of love.

I'm eighty-five years old. I've earned the right to indulge and break rules when I want to. Besides, this is my book...

And I know she's not *really* gone. Read on.

This is my truest, most vulnerable opportunity to memorialize her in the way she deserves, and I'm going to take full advantage of it.

So, on that note...

On Sunday, August 25, 2013, with members of our family and friends present, we unveiled Anna's beautiful gravestone. This was not a religious event, nor a sad one, but rather a celebration of her life and what she had meant to us.

I only cried briefly that day, for I instinctively knew and was comforted by the thought that we would actually speak again soon.

That day would come on December 30, 2013.

It has always been sad for me to walk through a cemetery and see so many gravestones identifying the people whose remains are there, but without any message as to who that person really was or what contribution they made to the betterment of society. Also, though I do consider myself a fairly religious man, I always felt it lacking somehow when a member of the clergy eulogized someone recently-deceased. Someone they never met. Sure, maybe the family filled them in, but for me, there's only one way.

And that way is to take matters into your own hands, just as I did when I instructed the funeral directors that Anna's stone was to be bronze with white flowers.

On December 30, 2013, as I walked towards Anna's site—passing many black and gray gravestones along the way—the tears that I held back on the day of her funeral began to flow.

The sun was shining, yet there was this one particular ray that seemed to be nipping at my heels. When I finally arrived at Anna's grave, after quite the walk, the ray hit the bronze stone and reflected off, shining upon me.

I was convinced that that ray was my beloved Anna.

My love...

This was the most incredible thing I have experienced in all of my eighty-five years. I told her about this book as I stood there sobbing for over an hour.

I promised her I would make her proud as her ray continued to shine, for we were, once again, speaking.

And, ever since, I have not feared death. Not at all.

Nor have I cried, because I know she is okay and that her spirit resides within me.

I will leave it at this. While Anna's spirit will forever live on in the hearts and minds of not only myself, but also, of course, our family and the many others who knew her, the message on her rose-colored stone with white flowers will forever commemorate the goodness and the fortune that she brought forth into this world.

ANNA PATRICIA OTIS

An Internationally Respected
Teacher Of The Blind
Adored By Her Husband And Family
And All Who Knew Her
1941—2012

I have been a very, very lucky man. To my sweet Anna, I will *always* love you...

———◆———

If there was a silver lining to any of my experience upon Anna's passing—and make no mistake, the death of a loved one is nothing to rationalize—it is that when she died when I was eighty-three years old, I was able to finally understand what others have told me in the past:

Tragedy brings good people together.

Acknowledgments

Several months after Anna's passing, while having lunch with our dear friend and Anna's primary caregiver Mimi Duca—who was provided by a wonderful company called Lifeline Companion Services—we were discussing all of the problems we encountered from my wife's initial diagnosis to the end of her life. Together, we formulated the idea of writing this book with the intent of helping others better prepare for their own inevitabilities.

Mimi continued to assist me in organizing and preparing the pages you are reading. As a professional caregiver, her keen insights have been invaluable to me.

I am most grateful for the help provided by Harold Bermudez, an executive of Leisure Care—a well-known, respected operator of retirement and assisted living facilities—and his excellent staff, without which I would not have had as easy access to much of the information regarding experiences with the dying and the elderly.

Joel Eisenberg, my longtime friend and book-writing expert, provided that extra push and encouragement and was always looking over my shoulders, as well as my publisher, Michael Conant, and my editor, Taylor Basilio, to ensure that I saw the big picture. Joel, Michael, and Taylor also spent hours organizing my words so that they made sense. I only hope their instincts were correct!

Family, for me, is a euphemism for fortune. In that event, I am also a very wealthy man. Thank you to my two sons, Ron and Rick, their wives, Judi and Leslie, and my daughter, Laurie, along with my five grandchildren and four great-grandchildren, and my step-son, David—all of whom have always been supportive of my efforts to do better (and also forgiving as I made bad judgements along the way).

My children inspired me as I watched them grow, and I've been further inspired as I've watched them raise their children to become caring and successful in their own right. Julie (and husband, Ben), Rebecca, Allyson, Ryan, and Jennifer (with husband, Scott), I love you.

I would be remiss if I did not acknowledge with deep gratitude the help, support and wonderful love given to me during the course of writing this book, by a group of dedicated friends. To Dr. Ron and Doreen Lever, Dr. Gordon Freeman, Michele and Michael Ginsburg, Dr. Jon Matthew, and my friend of over 75 years Dr. Fred and Sandy

Bernstein who along with Nooneh Kradjian, Ruth Goldman and Sherman Root gave me

the strength I needed to overcome the many obstacles that were placed in my path. I express my deep and abiding love.

And, finally (phew!), to my great-grandchildren, Noah, Addison, Tripp, and Caroline (a future star, who made her public debut on Facebook in December of 2013), you add the whipped cream on top of the cake.

I love you. Anna has loved you.

Life has been good.

So far…

Finally, I want to pay tribute to a man who up until almost his last day in December of 2014 was my mentor, friend, and inspiration. As you read this book, you will have an opportunity to learn about his teachings. Rabbi Harold Schulweis was in life as he is in death: A legend. That being said, I need to thank him posthumously for the difference he made in Anna's and my life.

A Tribute to a Legend

On Monday, September 30, 2012, I received a phone call from my dear friend and mentor, Rabbi Harold Schulweis, who advised me that he would not be attending Shabbat Services at our Synagogue, Valley Beth Shalom, in Encino, California, on the following Sabbath.

When I asked him why he told me that he was going to come to my home and spend that day with Anna. Since a long illness had left him weak and unable to drive, he asked me to pick him up and bring him to our home on Sabbath—which I did. He and Anna spent several hours alone with him holding her hand. She passed away one week later.

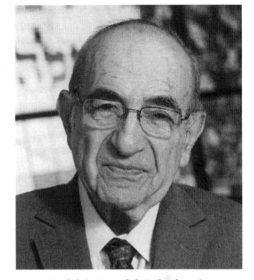

Rabbi Harold Schulweis

It is ironic that on the morning of October 18, 2014, just as I was just completing my final draft of this book, I received an e-mail advising me that the Rabbi had passed way earlier that day.

I would be less than true to his spirit if I did not acknowledge the part that this great Rabbi, author, and humanitarian played in my life, in addition to the contribution he made to people of all faiths and beliefs, as well as to this writing.

He read this book, contributed to its contents, and advised me as to the many concepts I have written about. Most of all, for close to thirty-two years, he and his beautiful wife, Malkah, were and are friends to Anna and myself.

I met him for the first time in 1983 upon my return to Los Angeles. It was following a difficult divorce and just before Anna and I met. I joined the Synagogue and sat with him to get his advice on my goals in life. He asked me if I was a good person.

My reply was that while I had made some mistakes in life, I felt that I was a good human being. He looked at me and told me to get up each morning, stand in front of a mirror, and applaud myself. I have done exactly that ever since.

Rabbi Harold Schulweis was and will be long remembered as a great scholar and teacher. Among his many contributions to those of all faiths was his founding of the Righteous Christians organization which paid honor to all those non-Jews who helped save so many Jewish lives during World War II.

His spirit resides in the hearts and minds of all of humanity.

My gratitude to him cannot ever be adequately expressed.

Contents

Preface

If young and middle-aged readers do not pick up this book, in addition to my own ancient demographic, then maybe I've wasted my time. I have to ponder that one a bit.

Here's the crux of the matter: Despite the looks, the jokes, the questions, the pity…I was young once too. Everything being well, you'll get there.

Here's the other crux: Serious illness and death are, unfortunately, not limited to the elderly.

If I'm doing my job as I hope (I'm eighty-five now, writing this from a retirement home and trying my damnedest), you will be provided with usable insight into the aging process, which I prefer to call *The Journey of Life*. This insight will allow you to not only properly plan for the future (if you are a younger reader), but if you are an older reader, it will also help you work through (the numerous) age-related issues.

Here is what I ask of you, regardless of your age:

Be open to new ideas; don't be stubborn. Learn from your mistakes. Share the wisdom of your wins. Remain an individual and contribute in ways only you can. Take reasonable risks. Listen more than you speak, and don't preach—you'll only alienate those you are trying to teach.

End the game on your terms.

Did I miss anything?

Anybody?

Well then…

I hope you enjoy my book. I trust (hope) that you will find my words highly informative and immensely inspiring.

Much like *The Journey of Life* itself, my book is a voyage with more twists, turns, trage-dies, and triumphs than any movie or novel could ever hope to capture.

If only it were so easy...

⤜◆⤚

Teach, Don't Preach

Allow me tell you a little story. I heard this once from a younger woman. She was around eighty-one at the time:

"So, Bernard—"

"Call me Bernie."

"So...Bernard. An elderly man—about eighty-seven, eighty-eight—was driving a large car down a busy highway with an eighty-three-year-old woman as a passenger. They were both very short and could not really see over the dashboard. You with me so far?"

"I'm with you."

"Mazel tov. When they approached a cross street, the driver went through a red light. The passenger didn't want to offend him, see, so she spoke to herself. You know what she said?"

"No idea."

"Didn't think so. She whispered to herself—the driver was a little deaf anyway, you know—'I think we just went through a red light. I sure hope I am wrong.' Still with me?"

"I'm still standing here, aren't I?"

"Standing? Trust me, not for long. Not without support, anyway…"

"No?"

"No. So, this driver and this passenger—and Bernard, please don't interrupt again—they came to yet another intersection. And the driver went through yet another red light. This time, the passenger thinks maybe she was imagining things, so she says nothing. She sits up as high as she can, though, and watches very closely. He does it again."

"Again?"

"Again! Bernard, please. So now she speaks up. She says to her driver friend, 'Do you know you've gone through three red lights?' And, Bernard, what do you think he said?

"I don't have the slightest—"

"He said, 'Are you suggesting that I'm driving?'"

I remember that day like it was yesterday. She laughed so hard she was rushed to the hospital, as she couldn't stop wheezing.

She *still* laughs. She's still around. And she repeats this joke to me every time I see her! Like she's never told me before! Yet, she laughs, she lives, she's happy.

There's a correlation there somewhere.

While I'm on the subject, I think it's a good time to address the *memory* issue for a moment. We'll get into it more later, but for now…

The memory slips a bit the older you get.

Surprised? I didn't think so.

Abraham Lincoln once said, "You cannot escape the responsibility of tomorrow by evading it today." While he may not have been speaking of old age, he may as well have been.

Confronting responsibility and planning for the future will be cornerstone topics of this book. You may as well get used to it now, as you may not remember your responsibilities in the future.

Note that I said may not, as opposed to will not.

Don't say I didn't warn you.

Thankfully, my memory is (still) intact. I say thankfully because when I consider my many reasons for writing this book, predominant among those reasons is that I'm doing this to honor my Anna.

She was full of vibrancy until her later years, when illness took hold.

And then I was alone. This was a new experience for me, as we were married for so long. On the day she passed, I was devastated. At her funeral, I celebrated her life.

And I realized that *I don't want to die with the music of life inside me.*

This is how my life changed upon Anna's passing. I want you all to know these intimate details first. This way, you can get to know and understand me as an individual, and I can reinforce to you that my circumstance is hardly unusual.

From there, we will get into the meat of this book: our A-Z voyage from birth to passing.

At 6:30 p.m. on a Thursday night in May 2010, the doctor who just performed an emergency appendectomy on Anna emerged from the operating room. The operation was a success; however, he proceeded to inform me that during the surgery they discovered a rare form of cancer in her system.

"Bernie…I'm sorry. She has less than two years to live," he said.

And that was that.

After absorbing this shocking news and asking the doctor a number of questions, I began my ride home in an obviously highly emotional frame of mind.

Over the next few hours and into the following days, three questions occupied my mind:

1. What did I need to do to ensure that Anna received the most informed medical care that was available?

2. What changes did I need to make in my life to ensure that I was always at her side during her treatment and care?

3. Who did I need to contact for information relative to finding a reputable home health-care agency that could provide us with assistance?

I wasn't ready. I wasn't prepared.

I needed help and learned quickly. I was lucky because I've had some relative experience. Not everyone does. Still, I couldn't help but ponder, if only I'd planned better...

Interestingly, the answers to all three of these questions were quickly provided, as I was able to use my many years of experience in dealing with the terminally ill, as well as the resources that were known to me. There was no question in my mind that all I had to do was remain calm and organized and our needs would be addressed.

The very next day, as Anna recuperated from the surgery, I met with my dear friend and primary care physician, Dr. Jonathan Matthew, who explained in detail what needed to be done medically. He, in turn, referred me to Dr. Omar Shaye and Dr. Ashkan Laskari, two well-known oncologists who gained my immediate confidence and proved the wisdom of that choice over the next two and a half years.

I began to slowly withdraw from my active career and devoted myself to being close to my beautiful and talented wife.

My cousins, Michelle and Michael Ginsburg, provided the answer to the third question when they introduced me to a person they had worked with in the home care industry.

Although, due to a financial drain caused by three recent family tragedies, we were not financially well-off, the one thing I was not concerned about was the cost of taking care of Anna; after all, we had one of the best health insurance and pharmaceutical plans available, along with what turned out to be one of, if not the best, long-term care programs. (If you do not have one, waste no time in finding one.) Fortunately for my professional life, my career and first book were doing well, which also eased the financial burden.

Though throughout my life I had worked as a volunteer caregiver—as something of a side career alongside my hospitality business—what I soon sadly discovered was that I (also) needed to now manage Anna's caregivers so she would get the best treatment possible. Before Anna's illness, I was able to go home at night and sleep off the occasional sadness. I always knew I was doing good work, caring for others and also regularly volunteering in hospices but—if you have a heart—the work does tend to affect you. Loss is never easy. And now I was home and could not take a break.

Caregiving for someone you love is, in itself, a full-time effort. The mental and physical strain of doing so can be incredibly intense.

Again, you must prepare for all possible outcomes.

It was during this difficult time that I, like so many others, forgot to check in with myself. Within three months, I had put on fifteen pounds, was sleeping five hours a night, and was just emotionally raw. I didn't know then what I know now: that caregiver burnout is real, and that the stress of caregiving comes on like a full-frontal attack.

In my case, my family and friends all told me that they could see the strain in my face. I sometimes I felt like I could barely breathe until Anna's ordeal was over. My best efforts were further complicated by difficulties with insurance companies and the daily long waits on hold, as well as mailing and faxing forms and documents which somehow continued to get lost in transmission.

Time passed. Anna became increasingly frail. And then...

She died.

That was it. Her *Journey of Life* was extinguished. To this day, I look back satisfied that I was able to be there for my beloved wife when she most needed me. If I have any regrets, it's that I was not well prepared. Again, to reiterate, I got lucky. I've been planning for the future ever since. And, by the time you finish reading, my greatest wish is that you will too.

Welcome to my book. May your journey, like mine, overflow with health, happiness, and most of all, love.

> "Father Time is not always a hard parent, and though he tarries for none of his children, he often lays his hand lightly upon those who have used him well; making them old men and women inexorably enough, but leaving their hearts and spirits young and in full vigor.
>
> With such people the grey head is but the impression of the old fellow's hand in giving them his blessing, and every winkle but a notch in the quiet calendar of a well spent life.
>
> —Charles Dickens

MY NAME IS BERNARD OTIS. WHAT'S YOURS?

Let's get to know each other, shall we?

Every good relationship begins with a first step.

A beginning.

So, the first thing you need to know about me is that I was born into a large Orthodox Jewish family in Detroit.

The second thing—which may be a result of my upbringing, who knows?—is that I've been told I have a rather bizarre sense of humor for an eighty-five year old.

How's this for size:

When Jason was told that his ninety-five-year-old grandfather had passed away, he immediately went to see his ninety-year-old grandmother to comfort her. When he arrived, he asked her what had happened.

The grandmother explained that her husband died while they were having sex.

Jason was stunned, and told his grandmother that he was shocked to find out that they were having sex at their age, suggesting that it was a "very bad situation."

The grandmother responded by telling him that she and the grandfather had discovered, a few years earlier, that if aging persons had sex when the church bells rang it was safe.

She said that it was all about the rhythm—that if you go in with the ding and out with the dong it was very relaxing and safe.

And then she added, "If that stupid ice cream truck hadn't come by, Grandpa would still be alive today."

Yay? Nay?

Okay. Onward...

We lived in a predominately Jewish neighborhood. We're talking an area that was about seventy-five percent Jewish, twenty percent Catholic, and the rest a mix of various religions.

My goal was to become an architect, an ambition I abandoned in my thirteenth year due to bad eyes. I did not attend the local high school (Central High), but instead chose to attend Cass Tech, a very well-known technical school that was located some seven miles from my home. I attended Cass Tech much to the chagrin of my parents who nonetheless allowed me freedom of choice. The streetcar and bus both got me back and forth except when there were transportation strikes, which was frequent.

In those dark times, I had to walk. I had no choice.

However, regardless of the occasional inconvenience, this decision—mine and mine alone—would prove to be a major turning point in my young life.

The student population of Cass Tech, a seven-story building in the downtown area of Detroit, was comprised of individuals seeking to become not only architects, but also artists, engineers, musicians, technicians, builders, chemical scientists...

They came from every race, creed, religion, ethnicity, financial level, and family status.

For the first time in my life, I was confronted with real options as to my future.

And a real mix of people that has enabled me in my lifetime to look upon everyone as an equal.

SENIOR MOMENT #1
TREAT EVERYONE AS AN EQUAL

Get used to these *Senior Moments,* by the way. I have a million of 'em.

Anyway, Cass Tech had a huge 3000-seat, civic-type auditorium that was often the center of visitation by world and community leaders. As president of the student council, it was my privilege to meet, dine with, and introduce them when they visited us.

Among those who I came to know and respect were Walter and Victor Reuther, the founders of the UAW-CIO, Senator Hubert Humphrey, Eleanor Roosevelt, and numerous others in every level of our society, including the most exciting and interesting Igor Sikorsky—one of the key designers and developers of the helicopter.

Yes, I knew Eleanor Roosevelt.

I told you I'm old.

Don't act so surprised.

But wait! There's more!

In 1946, in preparation of the automobile industry's fiftieth anniversary, my high school principal, Bill Stirton (later to become Dean of the University of Michigan), asked me to help coordinate a key component of a celebratory parade in downtown Detroit. I was assigned to work with baseball great Connie Mack and auto pioneer Henry Ford, both in their advanced years, to coordinate a food race down Woodward Avenue, Detroit's main street.

What an exciting learning experience for a teenager just getting his life started. All of this at a time when the Great Depression was winding down and the effects of WWII were changing our economy. In fact, while we did not realize it at the time, the stage was being set for the crisis we face today in our healthcare, cost of living, and education systems.

I'll be sure to address those issues shortly, I promise.

For anyone under the age of, say, fifty, you really have no idea how fast it (life) goes by. The preliminaries are already over. The days speed by when you hit that half-century mark. Trust me.

As Victor Hugo, author of *Les Miserables* and *The Hunchback of Notre Dame* once said, "Forty is the age of youth; fifty is the youth of old age."

He knew the deal. He got there too.

Allow me to add to his statement: "And every minute thereafter? A race against time."

I'm eighty-five as I write this. I need to finish this book. I need to keep up my blogs to promote this book. I need to maintain my consulting business, and most of all, I need to continue to meet my bills.

Just like you. Until I can no longer.

Regardless of your age, we're really are not all that different, you and I. I don't get through my day calling anyone "Sonny" either (one lasting stereotype I'll never understand).

Here's the rest of my reality: Though I'm eighty-five, I feel like I'm twenty-five. My mind and my heart is very much that of an average, red-blooded, American twenty-five year old. But the body...fuggetaboutit! (Did I tell you I was hip? Found that one in the Urban Dictionary, defined as "the Brooklyn way to say 'forget about it," originally used by Italian gangsters because of their funny accents.")

With apologies to Tony Soprano and the late, great James Gandolfini...

SENIOR MOMENT #2

TALK TO YOUR CHILDREN. THEY WILL APPRECIATE IT LATER ON

Enough of the games. Time to get down to business.

You knew it was coming.

At some point, I was going to have to get serious, and even a bit ugly. Aging isn't all that pretty, but the quality of your life is up to the decisions you make right now.

So, for my readers who have not yet touched that half-century mark, before you get here, know that you will soon enough, because why?

"T-I-M-E

G-O-E-S

F-A-S-T!"

Good job. You were paying attention.

So, before you get there, I would like for you to promise me you are going to strive for something more.

I call this one *A Victorious Journey*.

Cock your neck. Loosen up. Yesterday is over; it's time for a new day. Get the blood flowing (while you still can)!

Now, we're gonna work.

"I can teach anybody how to get what they want out of life. The problem is that I can't find anybody who can tell me what they want."

—Mark Twain

Many months ago, shortly after the passing of my beautiful wife, Anna, I went to sleep at my usual time: ten p.m. And then...the strangest thing happened.

I was a five year old living in Detroit, Michigan. Surely this couldn't be a dream; it was much too vivid. The sights, the sounds...I was back. Back to my childhood, back to a day that I recall now as being (mostly) happy and fulfilling:

I accompanied my father as he purchased a 1935 Plymouth for $750.00. A father-son bonding day. How I must have missed that as I traversed my reverie. My dad was thrilled, grinning ear-to-ear. (Hey, it's my book and my cliché; I'm almost eighty-six, what do you want?) He treated me to ice cream after and all was well in the world.

Later...

What a blast, I thought, as we drove home that night. I was certain that our entire family would be waiting at the front door to welcome us back from this perfect day, but my seventy-three-year-old Bubby (grandmother, in Jewish parlance) had fallen ill, and all of the aunts and uncles were at our home waiting for the doctor to arrive (in those days, doctors made house calls).

Back then, seventy-three was *really* old, and our neighborhood was filled with *really old people*. Many of these men and women were immigrants who had never learned to speak English, and by this point, most had memory problems, which were referred to as the sickness of age.

I could never understand why they could not hear what I said to them or why they gave me strange answers. Many of them could hardly walk.

There were few homes for the aged and most of these *really old people* lived with and were cared for by their families, and they were often kept in a bedroom hidden away from the rest of the world. And then, frequently, these neighborhood seniors seemed to suddenly disappear with alarming frequency.

"Ma?" I asked.

"Bernard?"

"What happened to Mrs. Lefkowitz?"

"Oh, Bernard..."

"Well...?"

"She died, Bernard."

"Died? What is 'died?'"

"We can't talk about that now. When you're a little older..."

"Can I ask you another question?"

"Bernard?"

"What happened to Mr. Bernescu? The camera store owner...? I haven't seen him in about two weeks—"

"Oh, he died two weeks ago."

"I don't understand."

"You will when you're older. You don't need to worry about such things now."

"Then what about Mrs.?"

"Bernard!"

After that conversation, I asked everyone I knew what "died" was. I finally learned, from a kind older man sitting on a street corner holding a tin can with some pennies, that the word I was looking for was death.

When I approached my mom after my impromptu lesson, she said, "Bernard, good for you. You have a curious mind and it will serve you well."

And that was that.

In fairness, most parents during that era stayed quiet on the subject.

I never quite understood. What were they protecting us from? God forbid that we young ones were told about such things as death at such a young age. And the statement that I didn't "need to worry about such things now?" How unfortunate. At the earliest age we need to let our children know about death and the important role it plays in our lives. It is a good word because it is real, and if we understand where it fits in our life's journey, that journey can be made a lot happier because our focus as we travel it will be to concentrate on making every day a happy experience.

By the way, I asked my dad, the sagacious one, the same question once I already found the answer. I figured Ma must have said something to him, but I really wanted to hear his response:

"Dad, what does 'died' mean?"

He furrowed his brow, deliberated over his response and finally said, "Read the funnies."

"But—"

"Trust me. You'll learn more about life and...otherwise...if you read the funnies."

My dad loved the funnies—the newspaper comic strips. He had a sense of humor. If he were still alive today, he'd still ask me to search the funnies for the answers to all of life's greatest questions.

Later on, at the age of fourteen after returning from my first funeral, I asked my father again. My father sat me down and opened up the Obituary section of the Detroit News. He said, "Son, I want you to look at each of these names and see what it says about their death."

He then pointed out numerous listings and read things like: "This man died from pneumonia," "this one from cancer," "this one had a heart attack." He said these were all the result of nature. By contrast, none of the obituaries said that a person died from hard work.

We wondered aloud how their families or friends helped them through the process.

So he said, "Son, always remember: Our main role in life is to help others create happy paths." He soon added, "But always make sure that your intent is true and not for gain, because no matter how pure and unselfish your intention may be, the person you wish to help could, for any number of reasons, find your motives self-serving."

Profound words which I remember to this day.

While we're on the subject, the following is a true quote from an eight-year-old girl: "When you die, God takes care of you like your mother did when you were alive—only God doesn't yell at you all the time."

Just thought I would share.

Moving on. Or, back, actually, to my dream.

The Great Depression was in progress and many of our family and friends were very poor. We often shared homes and food, and we made our own fun.

Here's an interesting dichotomy:

Today we live in a world of violent movies and videogames.

As time goes by, our society seems to have forgotten how much violence and killings were taking place at that time, the time of my childhood, due to the economic problems we were experiencing, as well as the growing religious hatred of that era.

My father was fortunate to have had a very good job in the food industry, which was going through a very difficult time due to the country being in economic struggle and also because some labor organizations were using murder and intimidation to get workers and businesses to join. I can still recall standing at the window of our home at six o'clock p.m. every night, my nose pressed against the glass, hoping that my father would return safely from work.

I said before, this was a mostly happy and fulfilling time for me, but it was also a very scary time for me.

As a result of my father's job, each Friday night our home was filled with poor relatives and friends. I watched with great interest as my parents handed out money and food that they had gotten through his work to them. He never would accept repayment, and when I asked him why, he repeated some words I will never forget (that I mentioned before):

"Help others create happy paths."

Suddenly, all was right in the world. Everything was so "right" and so "good" because both my mom and my dad were so generous that I realized just how special they were.

And, finally, I understood.

They weren't protecting me so much as ensuring I was raised as worry-free as possible, in a happy home, with good values. This way, as I got older, I could show others the way.

I didn't agree with everything, but I can see now how fortunate a child I was.

And then, suddenly, at the moment of my epiphany, I woke up.

The timing! I didn't want to leave the warmth of my parents' home. There were tears in my eyes. The memory of my parents, who passed on at such a young age, permeated my waking thoughts. I sat up in my bed, startled, and at that moment realizing that I was a *really old person* myself, as were most of my friends. I was no different than the other seniors I had been with when I was a young child.

And I started to cry...

SENIOR MOMENT #3

PRACTICE GOOD HEALTH SO YOU CAN REMAIN ACTIVE AND CREATIVE. "RETIREMENT" DOES NOT MEAN GIVING UP ON LIFE

When childhood passes, there is no need to feel sorry for yourself.

Grandma Moses began painting at eighty. Ronald Reagan did not become governor of California until he was sixty-one. Mahatma Ghandi became the leader of independent India as a senior citizen.

Charlie Chaplin, Clint Eastwood, and others directed films into their seventies and beyond. Frank McCourt, the author who wrote the worldwide bestselling memoir *Angela McCourt,* started writing in his sixties.

Leonardo di Vinci was drawing sketches in his sixties. Leo Tolstoy was writing novels into his seventies. Anthony Burgess of *A Clockwork Orange* did not start writing until he was in his forties. Michelangelo was sculpting into his eighties.

Marvis Lingren began running in her sixties and has competed all over the world for many years since. At 103 years old, Ben Levinsen set world records for the shot put at the Senior World Olympics.

Bernerd Herzberg completed a degree in his native German when he was over eighty years old. He had never before spoken the language.

And so it goes. Retirement did not come naturally to any of these achievers.

To them, I raise a glass of fine red wine—good for the blood pressure, you know—and dedicate the following double-header:

Okay, that was brief and concise.

I woke up, was old again after revisiting my youth, and felt sorry for myself. And then it passed.

Have *you* ever felt sorry for yourself? Did it pass? Of course it did—just like your youth will pass. Just like your adulthood will pass, and then one day...

This is a short chapter. Just like life. Point made.

SENIOR MOMENT #4

TIME FLIES. BE SURE TO MAKE
EVERY MOMENT COUNT

Therefore, my peeps (like that one?) to reiterate, predominantly, to my readers under fifty...

T-I-M-E

G-O-E-S

F-A-S-T.

They say us seniors don't remember anything, but I will repeat this one until *you* do.

T-I-M-E

G-O-E-S

F-A-S-T.

In that spirit, allow me to extend my hand in friendship to you, my reader.

Because you really don't know what you don't know until you know (try that one three times fast). You're in your prime! But believe me, you will later on.

And I've gained the wisdom to get you there in one piece.

A valuable benefit of being as old as dirt.

Ya got me?

The pithy among us state that a person begins to die the moment they are born.

You'll find a great deal of tongue in cheek humor in this book, but let's be real for a moment: Life is filled with challenges. It can be difficult, and it can break you down. You need to be strong. But, equally important, you need to be smart.

Cases in point:

Dr. Nancy Snyderman, the Medical Editor of "NBC Nightly News," told of her experience when she found herself having to take care of her aging mother and how, despite all of her years of reporting on medical issues, she was ill-prepared to deal with the outside problems related to her mother's aging.

"Caregivers tend to patients an average of twenty hours each week," she said, "but many would agree that it feels like more. Like me, about half are also balancing that responsibility with a full-time job."

Even though our insurance companies and governmental healthcare providers each year send us large books containing detailed information about our current coverage, it takes a Philadelphia lawyer to figure out the applicable interpretations of some of these rules and regulations—which is literally impossible.

Also, poor communication between doctors' offices and providers of medicines necessary for treatment frequently cause huge out of pocket expenses in order to avoid treatment delays.

And it goes on and on, as if it's not difficult enough to handle the impending death of a loved one...

⟫•⟪

During a recent interview I had with a retired eighty-nine-year-old professional, I asked him what he considered to be the biggest mistake he had made during his lifetime.

He told me that he deeply regretted not having spent more time developing personal relationships so as to avoid the loneliness he now felt—even though he has a lovely wife and family.

It is so sad to see elderly persons who have no close personal friends with whom to visit, share life's experiences with, and confide in.

Sort of reminds me of this old chestnut:

> An eighty-year-old man is sitting on a bench in Central
> Park. It is five in the afternoon and he is crying. A young
> businesswoman on her way home from work comes up to him
> and asks him what was wrong and why he is crying.
>
> He replies, "This is terrible. My first wife passed away one year ago
> today, and I remember I had such a hard time handling her affairs. Now
> I am married to a gorgeous blonde-haired, blue-eyed woman who takes
> very good care of me. She's as young as you. She cooks me wonderful
> meals and takes me out to dinners, theatre, and everywhere. She keeps
> a clean house and we enjoy a beautiful physical relationship."
>
> The woman is surprised and says: "So why are you crying?"
>
> He answers, "I cannot remember where I live."

In other words, love your loved ones and enjoy life (!) while you can. It goes quicker, much quicker, than you think.

According to The *New York Times*, nearly forty percent of Americans are caring for someone with a serious health issue. Those caretakers, the article goes on to state, are "likely to report poor health themselves and to shortchange their own financial futures."

In fact, there is a growing concern regarding the number of young and middle-age men and women who are no longer able to work full- or part-time because of the need to take care of their aging families.

What then?

Consider the words of this frightening report which appeared in The *Week* magazine on September 27, 2013:

"Two thousand, two hundred and fifty Americans were asked in a poll to pick an age at which they could live in good health forever. The average person's favorite age was fifty, when in fact it is at around that age that our minds and bodies begin an acceleration of aging issues and we should be heavily involved in planning the last phase of our life...though the average person, unfortunately, thinks otherwise.

While we would all look forward to a long and fruitful life, nature does has a way of disrupting the journey and shortening it through accidents, illness, birth defects, crime, war, terror, and so on. However, good things also happen to all of us and the totality of the life/death experiences should inspire us to find that joy.

Don't believe me? Read on

SENIOR MOMENT #5

LIFE IS NOT A BATTLE. IT IS A JOURNEY, AND IF YOU PREPARE EVERY STEP OF THE WAY, YOU TOO WILL BE VICTORIOUS

During my first year at the University of Michigan, I became enthralled with William Shakespeare's writing. In one of his most well-known plays, "As You Like It", he enumerates what he considers the Seven Stages of Life:

This wide and universal theatre
Presents more woeful pageants than the scene
Wherein we play in.
And all men and women merely players.
They have their exits and their entrances;
And one man in his time plays many parts,
His acts being seven stages. At first he is an infant
And then the whining school boy
And then the lover
Then a soldier
And then a Justice
The sixth stage shifts into the lean and slippered pantaloon with spectacles on nose
and pouch on side
Last scene of all,
that ends this strange and eventful history,
is second childishness and mere oblivion
Sans teeth, sans eyes, sans taste, sans everything.

These wise words ring as true today as when they were written, and they should be heeded by all of us as we plan our lives.

In the ensuing chapters of this book, we will look at each of these stages and hopefully capture an insight into the challenges we face with each.

As we do this, please keep the following in mind:

- Begin to plan the trip early in life and continually make adjustments to it as the aging process progresses.
- Always take into consideration the burden you will impose upon your loved ones during the process; this includes a decision to give up some or all of your independence.
- Whether you are faced with a life-threatening illness or just advancing age, do not be in denial. Work hard to maintain a positive attitude and speak openly to family and friends about any related issues you may have.

A 2013 article in the *Los Angeles Times* tells of a family whose religious faith dictated thusly: When they learned that one of the family members had a terminal illness, they instructed the sick man's medical caregivers, and all else who associated with him, to not tell him the truth. In fact, when he asked them why the treatment he was receiving did not to appear to be helping, they told him it was and that he would be fine.

How sad it is to deny a dying person the right to have a chance to make a choice about his or her own future, and to have the opportunity to live a quality of life to the very end. Even sadder is the continual denial of the dying person's right to say the appropriate goodbyes.

Here's a humorous yet sad true story:

On the occasion of their sixty-fifth wedding anniversary, Martha and David (names changed to protect the not-so-innocent), both in their late eighties were being interviewed by their local radio station. The reporter asked them, "If you had it to do all over again, would you have married each other?"

They both said, "Yes, without question."

"And if you had it to do all over again, would you have lived the same lifestyle?"

Again, they responded affirmatively.

"What about children? If you had it to live all over again, would you have had children?"

Without hesitation, Martha exclaimed, "Yes, but not the same ones."

Live! Plan! Age! Live!

Until you're *kaput*. Hopefully, you have quite a while before you go *kaput*.

Huh?

Trust me on this.

Let's get into it, shall we?

LIVE!

If I need to explain this one to you...

Okay, okay. I won't assume anything from here forward. I can be a bit of a wise guy (actually, I've been called worse), but we have legitimate business to attend to.

I have a good friend whose father passed away at the relatively young age of seventy. They were as close as father and son could be. My friend has two brothers and his mom is, thankfully, healthy.

His dad always used to say, "Life goes so fast. Wherever did the years go?"

Just like me.

There will come a time—usually this happens, statistically, at about fifty years old for most people—where you realize that, suddenly, you are moving towards the last phase of your life.

From here, generally, comes a veritable speedway of regret; of rushing; of planning your bucket list.

So how do we combat this sudden bout of the "oh darns?"

Live!

Live a rich and fulfilling life, and live out your years as happy and healthy as you possibly can. Obstacles will come and obstacles will go. Make your ride as worthwhile as worthwhile can be.

To do this best of all, however, be sure to also incorporate the following:

- If your family lives far away, in your plans be sure to incorporate your friends and/or religious affiliations and/or organizations and/or... You get the picture.
- Always include your caregivers or medical professionals in the loop, as they will need to know your points-of-contact should something happen.
- Also, make it an ongoing practice to read as many articles on this subject as you can, and keep yourself well informed about all related issues.

PLAN!

As good health is a key to good living...

From the earliest age possible, all adults need to prepare a health care plan that clearly defines what their wishes are should they become seriously ill or have an unfortunate event happen that effects their longevity.

Either may well happen in your lifetime.

Your plan should include the following:

A Legal Advanced Health Care Directive. The LAHCD will indicate who you wish to make decisions for you in the event of personal incapacitation, and it should:

a) Include a statement as to what minimal quality of life you will accept when end of life decisions are made; and

b) Clearly define who, in descending order, is to be responsible for making decisions on your behalf. Note that said person should be close to where you live. Both you and every family member need to discuss and agree as to *who* is responsible for *what* in case of a serious illness. This process must continue and be updated on a regular basis. In the event of differences of opinion, you might want to hire a knowledgeable professional to help in this process.

When planning one's health needs in the future, keep in mind that long-term health insurance is extremely costly. A well-qualified financial planner is a must in this process.

Harold Bermudez, the General Manager of a major Southern California health care living center, recently told me of his greatest concern. This concern is that, over the next several years, the average income of most Americans will, again, be significantly decreased. Costs for such world events as the Iraq war, for example, must finally be paid for and will ultimately result in yet another deleterious hit in the wallet.

Bermudez expects a financial hailstorm that will, once again, effect our ability to be financially able to enter into long-term health facilities and will also increase the pressure on family and close friends to help find a way to care for the aged in their own homes.

Allow me to return, for a moment, to your LAHCD:

c) You must include a complete, easy-to-access medical history file with records of medical tests and medications (including ones that do not work for you). Be certain that you and your family discuss and document the family's medical history as well.

d) Document your funeral desires and/or preferred plans.

e) Invest in a Long Term Care Policy early in your life. It could be the best investment you can make.

AGE!

Follow the above instructions and you will free yourself from an immense amount of stress later, because less stress later will help you age gracefully.

And do not hesitate to have social relationships younger than yourself. Age should not restrict how you live a happy life. Onward and upward.

DEATH.

It'll happen, folks.

In that spirit (that was bad, wasn't it?), I am looking most forward to meeting you, my readers, on the other side. We'll rendezvous at my first book signing in Heaven, address forthcoming.

But remember to live first. I gave you the roadmap. The rest is up to you.

The rest.

SENIOR MOMENT #6

THE SENSE OF SIGHT AFFECTS ALL THAT WE DO

Said the little boy, "Sometimes I drop my spoon."
Said the old man, "I do that too."
The little boy whispered, "I wet my pants."
I do that too," laughed the little old man.
Said the little boy, "I often cry."
The old man nodded, "So do I."
"But worst of all," said the boy, "it seems
Grown-ups don't pay attention to me."
And he felt the warmth of a wrinkled old hand.
"I know what you mean," said the little old man.

—Shel Silverstein, *The Boy and the Old Man*

The importance of the senses—sight, in particular—cannot be understated. Have you ever walked into a room filled with people or gone to a meeting and immediately had a view of those gathered there that instinctively allowed you to sense, see, and feel the mood and energy level that existed in that setting?

All too often we are incapable of recognizing that which is right before our eyes. Parents are so busy trying to earn a living, raise and educate their children, and even caring for their aging parents that they don't stop long enough to see what concerns their young ones have.

Our aging parents are unwilling to recognize that they have mobility and other physical problems that could put them in danger. They don't see that they need to give up their independence and begin to rely on others.

And even sadder is how often all parties do see the obvious but will not share their fears with each other. Just think of this: One of the largest causes of death amongst those sixty years or older is complications from falls in their own homes.

What precautions have you and your loved ones taken to protect yourself from the danger you are putting yourself in by refusing to see the obvious? Have you and your loved sat down to talk about these issues in an honest, forthright way?

It is never too early to learn how to go about making your advanced years comfortable and safe. You will discover that along the road which we travel—from birth to death—there are many not-so-obvious danger zones that we had better start looking for and planning around early on.

I recall as a young child living in Detroit, one of our family's big joys was riding from our home in the Northwest section of the city to Belle Island, which is located many miles away. (There were no freeways at that time.) We traveled on the Detroit River across from Windsor, Ontario, Canada.

Although I have not visited it for many years, at that time it was a place that had all kinds of winter and summer activities including water sports, boating, ice skating and fireworks on the river.

There was also a large outdoor music amphitheater that featured well-known personalities. I was most impressed and intrigued by the great Leonard Bernstein who performed there often.

While my family loved his performances, I was glued to his music methodology. He always moved his arms and legs so harmoniously and seemed to have mystical look on his face.

When I mentioned this to others they said they did not notice those things because they were concentrating on the music. I have never forgotten that intrigue and several years later, following his death, there was a major article in the *New York Times* speaking about Leonard Bernstein (I regret not having kept it) in which a music critic wrote that few people noticed that the thing that set Mr. Bernstein apart from others and made him such a master was the total involvement of his physical and mental being as he led the orchestra.

How much time do we spend watching our friends and loved ones as they involve themselves in life? Do we really absorb the way our aging parents handle their lives, or are we so happy to see them get through every day that we fail to see how unhappy they are in doing so?

Are we so busy doing things that we don't take the time to take a step back and actually see and *feel* the emotions that are involved in our everyday living? I think not.

The owner of a large American furniture manufacturing company
went to Hungary to purchase some materials for his company.

As he was leaving a restaurant, he passed a very beautiful woman
who smiled at him. He returned the smile and attempted to make her
acquaintance but because of the differences in their languages.

He drew a picture of a car and she indicated
agreement, so they went for a ride in his car.

He drew a picture of a bar and she nodded in agreement, so
they went to a bar and had a few drinks. He drew a picture of
two dancers, so they got on the dance floor and danced.

She then indicated that she wanted to use his paper and
pencil and she drew a picture of a four-poster bed. He was
confused and dropped her off where this had all started.

The next day he was telling a friend about his experience with the woman
and said, "I wonder how she knew I was in the furniture business?"

Not long ago I walked through an assisted living center with the family of a woman with Alzheimer's disease who had just been admitted. As we walked along, one of the persons in our group pointed out the beautiful furniture, the lovely dining room, and the precious paintings on the wall.

"Oh, what a beautiful place in which to live" she exclaimed. I asked her "What about the people, the residents? Do you think they see it as you do?" She was absolutely speechless as she suddenly realized that we were surrounded by men and women who had no feelings, were lost in their own world, and for whom Buckingham Palace or the back alleys of New York would be the same.

Nothing gets me more upset than to hear families tell me that I must see the lovely place they have chosen as the home for their aging a parents, or the beautiful school they are sending their children to.

What has that have to do with the poor quality of life I see them living, or the manner in which parents treat their school-aged children by using the beautiful school as a baby sitter?

A member of my family is a devoted schoolteacher who lives some miles from my home. She also has a physical disability that makes driving long distances difficult. I am often driven to see her, as happened not long ago.

It was after hours and she had classroom preparations to make for the next day so we met at her school and spoke as she worked late into the day.

Outside of the school building there were many young elementary-age students running around unattended, throwing dirt balls at each other, screaming, shouting, etc.—all of this on the grounds of a beautiful school in an upscale neighborhood.

"Why?" I asked. The answer to what I saw was that their parents had not yet come to pick them up.

Are we so blind to the needs of so many? Do we not want to see how we are failing to understand and address the real issues that deny those who depend upon us even a slightest bit of happiness?

Yes, my dear friends, we do need to take a step back and not only see what is going on around us, but to understand it and take positive steps to letting those we love flounder in what we see as beautiful surroundings.

> "The relation between what we see and what we know is never settled.
> Each evening we see the sun set. We know that the earth is turning away
> from it, yet the knowledge, the explanation, never quite fits the sight."
>
> —John Berger, *Ways of Seeing*

When my granddaughter, Julie, graduated from the University of Austin, Texas, I jokingly told her that she needed to get a good job so she could take care of me as I got older. Julie quickly responded, while laughing,

"That's my father's job."

She was right. I laughed. But then I thought about it some more.

How did it all start? When did I start getting...old? Who really is supposed to take care of who, here?

Looking back, at least in my case, I see that it all started with a warning. But we'll get to that later. I want to be more general first.

As the aging process proceeds, there are often signs of possible serious problems ahead, which both we and our loved ones try to ignore and treat as if they are just normal to our lives. In fact, if quickly and seriously acted upon, loved ones can help minimize and/or eliminate the problem before it becomes a major issue.

My dear friends, Doctors Ron Reider and Judi Freir, were discussing the importance of the five senses to a small audience of lecture-attendees. Suddenly, Ron called our attention to a biblical commentary that said that while all senses were important, *seeing* had one major additional benefit that the others lacked.

When the group asked what that was, Ron indicated that it was the ability to see and retain a fuller view of the issues. For example, you can look into a crowd of people and see someone who attracts your attention, and we can look at a piece of art and become emotional about it. We can go to a mountaintop and view the beauty of the valleys, etc.

While attending a business event at a California resort in 1983, I looked across the dining room and saw my wife-to-be, Anna, for the very first time. It was an immediate feeling of love at first sight.

What better example can I provide than the poem my friend and mentor, Rabbi Harold Schulweis, a legend in the Jewish Rabbinate, wrote about the famous Violinist, Yitzhak Perlman, in his "Playing with Three Strings."

> "We have seen Yithak Perlman
> Who walks the stage with braces on his legs
> On two crutches
>
> He takes his seat, unhinges the clasps on his legs,
> Tucking one leg back, extending the other,
> Laying down his crutches, placing the violin under his chin.
>
> On one occasion one of his violin's strings broke,
> The audience grew silent but the violinist did not leave the stage.

He signaled the maestro, and the orchestra began its part,
The violinist played with power and intensity on
Only three strings.

With three strings he modulated, changed and
Recomposed the piece in his head
He re-tuned the strings to get different sounds,
Turned them upward and downward.
The audience screamed with delight,
Applauded their appreciation

Asked later how he had accomplished this feat,
The violinist answered
It is my task to make music with what remains.

A legacy mightier than a concert,
Make music with what remains.
Complete the song left us to sing,
Transcend the loss
Play it out heart, soul and might
With all remaining strength within us."

What a beautiful way to live out our lives until death do us part.

We live life as a performer, in front of our audience. We see our audience as they see us.

Our family and those close to us are the major parts of our audience. We can all see symptoms which tell us that our loved ones are having problems which need to be addressed, but we keep our eyes closed and pretend that it is not happening. We need to attend the concert so that we can applaud the result.

While writing the opening to this chapter, I spoke to a woman who asked me if I knew of someone who could move into her ninety-three-year-old father's home in exchange for room and board. She said she needed someone to take care of him.

When I explained to her the legal and other ramifications of not hiring a trained licensed caregiver to do that, she replied, simply, "He is not ready for that yet."

How can we not see that a person that age is beyond ready?

The importance of the sense of *seeing* becomes more apparent as we realize that if we keep our eyes open and not be in denial, we will easily see signs of possible aging problems and act upon them.

THE SIGNS OF AGING:

1. Confusion and unusual behavior

   Caregivers should stay calm and try to determine the cause of this behavior.

2. Sudden loss of temper including shouting and hollering

   The person may be in pain, have been challenged by brain damage, feel lonely and afraid, bored, concerned about their failing memory, or be irritated by too much noise.

   If they are calling out to someone from their past try to speak to them about that to calm them down. In any event, you should consult with their primary care physician about these issues.

3. Repetitive questioning, unusual actions or movements

   Boredom and the need for more contact with others may be the reason for this. This could be the result of any number of things including, stress, a noisy environment, discomfort, etc.

   Be certain that the individual is not too hot, cold, hungry, thirsty, or constipated. It would also be wise to contact the primary doctor to ascertain if there are some pain or medication issues.

4. Dementia

   - Hiding and losing things
   - Pestering people and making persistent phone calls
   - Instability and falling
   - Night-time walking
   - Forgetfulness and irritability

Many or even all of these issues could be related to Alzheimer's or other advancing age conditions which, if looked into and acted upon early, can make it possible to deal with in a calm manner—rather than waiting for them to become difficult to resolve.

It is important if you live on your own (or even with members of your family) that all of those close to you know about and discuss these issues and not act as if everything is okay.

Also, as we get older, we need to make certain that the environment in which we live is made as safe as possible. When you consider that one in three individuals over the age of sixty-five falls every year, and close to seventy percent of accidental deaths of senior citizens is a result of a fall, you realize how serious a problem this is.

Falls result in death or a higher likelihood of the need to enter a care facility, major hip damage, and the onset of all kinds of life-threatening illnesses among seniors, as well as loss of mobility.

Again, look and *see*. The signs of aging are nothing to ignore.

FALLING

The Center for Disease Control estimates that the costs associated with falls by seniors is twenty-seven billion annually, and by the year 2020 will exceed forty-three billion.

The following is a list of actions that should be taken to minimize the chances of having a life-threatening fall:

1. Install Grab bars, commode extenders, non-slip bath mats, tub bench or bath chairs, and handheld shower attachments in your bathroom.

2. Remove all throw rugs from your home. They are dangerous.

3. Be sure that all clutter, including protruding electrical cords, are cleaned up and that all areas where you walk are free of hazardous situations.

4. Make sure that all stairways are safe and that stairs are marked with reflective tape to make navigating them as easy as possible.

5. Use night lights in all rooms.

6. Be certain that all chairs, including those on casters, are sturdy and safe to sit on and stand from. Bar stools and old kitchen chairs are of particular concern.

7. High bookshelves are dangerous and things that you regularly reach for on them should be on the lower shelves.

8. Avoid wearing long, flowing robes and floppy slippers which one can easily trip on.

Carefully consider using a cane, but be very selective when doing so. Be certain it is very sturdy, at the right height, and easily balanced. Not all canes are made for the needs of the aged.

An important note: If you have recently begun taking drugs for high blood pressure, you might have an increased risk of falling and fracturing your hip due to dizziness and/or fainting when standing. Call you doctor immediately if you experience such conditions.

Keep in mind that aging persons who are admitted to the hospital for pneumonia have a high risk, after being discharged, of challenges from loss of memory, falling, and depression, among other things, and may have future need to be admitted to nursing homes and other care facilities.

During the process of writing this book, I have spoken to individuals, families of the aged, doctors and others who have been hospitalized or spent time in various facilities due to an illness or a fall, and they have all told me that following the return home, many or all of the aforementioned symptoms have occurred.

It would appear that inactivity during the hospitalization and recovery period has many ramifications as we age.

SENIOR MOMENT #7

DON'T DIE BEFORE YOU HAVE TO

Death. Do you need me to tell you it doesn't get more serious than this, folks?

I didn't think so.

You're still young but don't ignore the subject. Huge mistake. Here's the big misconception, though, about dying: Death does not only come to those who stop breathing—death comes to those who stop living. Those who stop being happy.

As Frank Bures of The Rotarian said, in his wonderful article entitled "The Rewards of Risk-Taking" (January 2013):

"What's the greatest threat to the pursuit of happiness? Doing nothing. "

In his inspiring article, Bures tells the story of Dave Freeman, an author who wrote a series of books about life, including *100 Things to Do Before You Die* which encouraged people to plan their life and get out and experience new adventures. He said, "This is a short journey, so get off your butt and create a fabulous memory or two before it is over."

Dave had an accident and died at the age of forty-one.

But he *lived* in the meantime. *Lived* deliberately in italics.

Though Freeman, sadly, who had a long list of things he wanted to do in his life, was only able to accomplish half of his plan, he did so with grand motivation and moxie.

> "Ah, great it is to believe the dream,
> As we stand in youth by the starry stream,
> But a greater thing is to fight life through,
> And to say at the end, the dream is true."

While most persons think of aging and death as something that persons in their late sixties and up have to be concerned about, the fact is that every day we learn about illnesses, accidents, and other situations that cause the death of young persons.

Consider this: Charles was a seventeen-year-old high school student who had his college plans made and a career in engineering planned when he was diagnosed with cancer of the pancreas following a period of excruciating pain. He died less than one month later.

Sammy was twenty-five-year-old podiatrist who was killed in an automobile accident. Mike was working his way through college when he was shot and killed during a robbery. And on and on.

How many times do we learn about young athletes who are seriously injured or killed doing what they most like to do? Are there any better reasons for families to openly speak about life's travails and also to discuss death? I think not. Life's too short.

Planning (that dreaded *P-word* again; I warned you) for both the expected and the unexpected is a must.

This certainly does not in any way suggest that we must walk around sad and afraid because these things could happen to us, but rather we should include them as matter-of fact life situations, which, as the years go on, can certainly effect us. Or, our friends, relatives, etc.

Here's a little ditty; a perfect example of a woman who *lived...*

"A woman in her late-nineties needs some birth control pills. The doctor is obviously surprised and asked her why she thinks she needs them. She tells him that they help her sleep better. "I don't much like sleeping but I need to be rested for my days." The doctor asks her how birth control pills help her sleep better. She tells him, "I don't take them, but I put them in my granddaughter's coffee each morning and that helps me sleep better."

But it's not yet over. He asks, "Is that why you look so good? Because of your sleep?"

"No. That would be because I have four boyfriends."

"You're kidding me."

"Nope. I begin each day with Will Power, and then go for a walk with Arthur Ritis. I usually return home with Charlie Horse and spend the evening with Ben Gay."

SENIOR MOMENT #8

ALTHOUGH IT IS BEST TO LET OTHERS BE THE JUDGE OF YOUR CHARACTER, IT IS EQUALLY IMPORTANT TO LOOK INWARD AND EVALUATE YOUR OWN ACTIONS WHEN HELPING OTHERS. THIS WAY, YOU WILL STAY TRUE TO YOUR EFFORTS

Very early in life we find that there are things we *want* to do, and other things which we try to avoid but which we *need* to do. My experience has been that whenever a *need to* occurs, such as going to a funeral, visiting a sick friend, getting up and going to work, or even a mundane task such as doing the dishes, if you think hard about it and find some good reason(s) why doing so would be of benefit to not only the recipient, but to you as well, if you change your attitude and make it a *want to*, you will find your life much less stressful.

Marian has a son who lives with her. At seven on a Tuesday morning, she called out to him that it was time to get up and go to school.

He hollered out, "I do not want to go to school. I don't like the teachers. The food in the cafeteria is terrible. And the students are very immature and mean."

Marian called back to him and said, "But you have to go to school. You're the Principal."

Allow me to be serious for a moment, shall we? Only by openly speaking about life and death, and planning the steps of the trip will you find life's journey worthwhile. So share your thoughts and dreams with your loved ones, read about the experiences others have had, maybe get some smiles along the way, and—

What?

"Too repetitive," you say? You know, that's the problem with you under-eighties today; you kids have no patience.

No matter. I'm moving onward with some real inspiration, where need tos and want tos are one, and positive perspectives prove that happiness is the only way to go.

CASE STUDY #1

A close member of my family is in her mid-nineties, and, with the exception of a bad back which affects her walking, she is as active physically and mentally as a much younger person.

During her lifetime, she has been challenged by more tragedy than anyone could imagine, including the loss of her mother early in life, a child shortly after birth, the death of her husband when she was in her late-forties and the losses of a host of companions along the way.

Nevertheless, following her periods of mourning, she has always maintained a happy attitude and enjoyed life. Her two daughters, who she raised alone by opening a successful catering company, are loving and kind and absolutely adored by all.

Ruth is upbeat every hour of her life and believes that when her time comes, her spirit will be warmly received and rewarded in the world to come.

Throughout it all, she certainly didn't *need to* be upbeat. She *wanted to* be upbeat.

She *chose to* be upbeat.

CASE STUDY #2

In 1978, my close friend and mentor Nathan Adelson—a founder and Executive Director of Sunrise Hospital in Las Vegas where I ran a division of a major corporation in the food and beverage facility design, planning, and grocery industries—was diagnosed with terminal cancer.

The end was near and would ultimately prove but months away.

So what did my friend *want to* do?

When his family and friends asked him what he wanted as a memorial to his life, he told them that he wanted a hospice program set up in his name. As a result, The Nathan Adelson Hospice in Las Vegas was established.

Many years later—2013, in fact—the Small Business Institute for Excellence in Commerce would name the Nathan Adelson Hospice the winner of its 2013 Nevada Award for Excellence.

While I had been involved in helping those in need for many years—through my work in Rotary and other similar organizations—I joined with this group in 1979 in honor of my late friend and received my first formal training as a hospice caregiver.

It never occurred to me at that time that my hands-on experience as a caregiver would, over the next thirty-five years, not only add so richly to my life, but also prepare me for the tragedy of losing my beautiful wife, as well as the events that have followed.

My sarcastic sense of humor aside, as you progress in this book you will understand why, at a very young age, I began to realize how helping others should become the foundation of my moral beliefs (even as I readily admit that my own failures have at times caused them considerable pain; in the interest of honesty, we will get to that as well).

CASE STUDY #3

This one is about me.

On November 21, 1980, a fire at the MGM Hotel in Las Vegas killed eighty-two people. During that tragic event, the Nathan Adelson Hospice was called upon to provide volunteers to help with the various issues that had to be addressed.

At the request of the person in charge of our staff that evening, my assignment was to station myself at the county morgue to handle the process of identifying the victims and contacting their families.

It was frightening to speak to so many young people who had been left with babysitters and no close relatives, thousands of miles from where their parents were supposedly having a great time, and having to inform these youngsters that they would never see their parents again.

Fast-forward thirty-four years.

So, why would an eighty-five-year-old man living in an assisted living center *want* to spend his time writing a book that at times revisits such tragedy, while continuing to work in this profession as well as helping others...all these years later?

Because that is my *choice*. This is what I *want*.

I'm actually asked this question quite a bit.

The rest of my answer?

Because I am still alive and have not achieved all of my goals. And, within my moral code, I have been taught to repent for my own transgressions and plant the seeds of which those who follow can harvest.

Period.

Life Authenticated

Helping others in an effort to attain personal praise is disingenuous at best. It is dishonest and harmful at its worst.

For those young ones reading this book, allow me translate:

IT SUCKS!

Understood?

> "There is one elementary truth, the ignorance of which kills countless ideas
> and splendid plans; the moment one definitely commits oneself, then Prov-
> idence moves too. All sorts of things occur to help one that never
> otherwise would have occurred.
> Whatever you can do,
> or dream you can do,
> begin it.
> Boldness had genius, power and magic in it.
> Begin it now."

—Goethe

Like Goethe said, "Begin it now." What did he mean by that?

He meant, "Begin *living* now." Which, by extension, means one must be prepared. To prepare oneself leads to a life authenticated, as referenced in our chapter heading.

And, what does *life authenticated* mean?

It means living an honest life, not a disingenuous one. I know, I know. There goes that repetition again.

One of the key characteristics of some of the world's great leaders has been that they have, most of their life, been surrounded by family, friends, business associates and acquaintances who have not only filled them with love and respect, but from whom they have been able to learn and translate that warmth into a wealth of leadership and knowledge.

Such has been my own unsolicited reward for which my gratitude overflows.

At the start of this book I wrote that from the moment we are born, aging and death are two certainties of life and we need to fear neither, but rather prepare for the journey and understand how, by doing so openly, our trip will be exciting and challenging.

There is a biblical story that suggests that the world was created three times. The first was a world of evil and that did not work. Then it was recreated with only good things and that did not work either, so it was finally created to contain good and evil and mankind was left to sort that out.

Why? So we learn our lessons and understand the difference.

During my research for this writing I found an interesting commentary by Rabbi Joseph Telushkin in his tome, *Jewish Wisdom*, a collection of...Jewish wisdom. (How long did it take you to figure that one out?) Quoting the analysis of Yalkut Shemoni as it regards Ecclesiastes 968: "If God didn't conceal from each person the day of his death, there would be no one to build a house, or plan a vineyard; each person would think rather, *Tomorrow I will die. Why should I work for others?*"

Thus, according to this fairly literal analysis, God concealed the day of a person's death so that he will build and plant. If he merits a long life, he will enjoy the fruits of his labor.

I ask you, regardless of your religious beliefs or lack thereof: What better way to look at life and strive to live each day so as to feel a sense of accomplishment, and know that we are at the same time making a brighter future for those who follow us?

I agree fully with that passage. *That* is what life is all about.

That, and hope.

Hope is of the utmost necessity. Hope for a better tomorrow. Hope for the end of challenges and pain (though neither physical impediment nor age should ever become an excuse to lose hope). Hope for a happy journey through life. Plan to attain that hope. We only fail when we stop trying.

So, all that being said, what is the moral of this chapter?

Practice everything that has passed to this point, in this book, and you too will have attained the joy and validation of an authenticated life.

SENIOR MOMENT #9

THE GREATEST MYTH OF ALL—
"I DID IT ALL BY MYSELF"

During my lifetime, I have had the privilege of meeting and receiving advice from some of the greatest business, religious, educational, and political leaders of the world.

In 1957, as President of the Harper Woods, Michigan Rotary Club, I was thrilled to be able to introduce our guest speaker, S.S. Kresge, the famous retailer who founded the "dime stores" bearing his name. These stores later became K-Mart.

I asked him what advice he would give to a twenty-eight year old like me who was just moving up in his career. His response was interesting. He said, "Young man, if you want to live with the classes, learn to deal with the masses and build good relationships."

As I look back over my life and watch what is happening in our world, this advice seems so pertinent, even in today's world. Each time I hear someone say. "That he is self-made," or, "They did it on their own," I think to myself, "Really? Are you saying their parents or teachers didn't wisely or wrongly influence them? Did their many friends and relatives not add to their thought process? Was their ability to finance their success free of financial institutions and institutions?"

I think, "Was their success not made possible through the help of employees and vendors? What about the love and support they received from their partners, children, and others in their lives? And finally, when illness, tragedy, and/or the aging process struck them, was their continued success luck or did others step in to continue what they'd started?"

Join me on a tour of life. Visit the many enterprises I have visited, meetings I have attended, trade shows that I have been involved in, and most importantly, go to the hospitals, rehab centers, private homes, and visits to the elderly with me.

Speak with the many single, young mothers who have been left alone and with the task of raising and supporting their families who, in the course of doing so, have come up with innovative business ideas.

I recently had met such a person. Denise is beautiful, dynamic, personable, energetic, and very positive about life. She came upon a water filtering system that produced healthy, clean water and decided to start a distribution company to promote its use.

She asked me if I would allow her to demonstrate it to me, and I agreed. Because of my marketing/sales expertise, I was more fascinated with her dedication and determination to be successful than I was about the excellent idea she had. Following the presentation, we discussed that, and I shared some ideas with her on how to succeed.

Ask all of those whom I have described if they could have done it on their own.

What is the point of all of this? It is that in every phase of our lives, we need others to help us. Whether in business or education, it's important to recognize that as much as we do not want to become dependent on others as we grow older, we do and we will.

We are not born as individuals. We are born into a community of persons, and if we are to have a happy life, overcome adversity, and achieve the success of a happy life, then we need to build relationships, help each other, and be willing to accept others' help from an early age.

There is a story told about a very successful industrialist who was being introduced as a featured speaker at a New York banquet. The person introducing him made a point of saying that the speaker had come to the United States from Europe many years before carrying his belongings in a sack tied to the end of a long pole and had gone on to build an empire.

Following the guest speaker's address, a man walked up to him and asked, "What was it you were carrying in that sack on the end of the pole?" The speaker sheepishly replied, "$25,000 in cash and a million dollars in stocks and bonds."

While it would be nice to believe that every successful person was so well endowed when they start out, the fact is that vision and smart work habits are just part of the success formula. Other people are a necessary ingredient, and that is why it is so important to always work on developing relationships with others.

In the early 1920s and 30s there was an Italian family of immigrants who operated a small chemical company in Detroit Michigan. The family had been doing so on a very small scale for many years, actually producing their product in a bathtub-type environment and selling it to households and businesses.

It was during the Great Depression, and financially, the company was struggling. My father, an accountant (before there were CPAs) managed a well-known meatpacking firm for a Catholic family whose owner was dying of Cancer. The owner of the chemical company was a customer of the chemical company.

One day the owner came to my father and told him that his company was in trouble and needed $3000 or they would go out of business. I witnessed this conversation even though I was just a young boy.

The owner of the chemical company offered to give my father a fifty percent interest in the firm in exchange for the money. Dad told him that he was not in the business of investing in other firms, handed the man $3000, and told him that he should not worry about repayment—just be successful.

The name of the product was Roman Cleanser. For those who do not remember it, think Clorox!!!

It may sound good to talk about doing it on your own, but behind every successful man is not only a nagging wife (ha-ha), but also a friend who understands.

It is not my intent in writing this to dwell on celebrity and flash famous names, but rather to share the stories of real people doing good things to reach out to help others. By doing so, it demonstrates that we all need each other and we cannot do it on our own as a community or as an individual.

A relative of mine was a very well-known executive in the entertainment industry who worked hard and with much help achieved fame and fortune for himself and his family. In fact, his wife's family was so poor that relatives had to help them survive.

Every weekend he would take his children out in his convertible, place hundreds of dollars in large bills on his sun visor, and drive through the poorest neighborhoods of Los Angeles handing those bills to homeless individuals gathered on street corners.

When asked why he would give large sums of money to total strangers who might use it for the wrong things, he responded by saying it was not his place to tell others how to spend their money. He said that they deserved the opportunity to have a chance at life and decide on their own the route they would take.

No matter what your financial status, education level, race, or religious beliefs, it is vital that every member of a community find a way to help another person. Whether with money, food, encouragement, or a work opportunity help and support should be happily given. The only repayment that you should hope for is love and seeing the success that comes from it

SENIOR MOMENT #10

DON'T EVER GIVE UP. CHOOSE LIFE

Let's say you are a teenager. You're dating, going to school, having fun, stressing...and you dream one night of meeting someone with whom you will fall in love and grow old with.

Sleep happens, and then the reverie. You find this book, you come to this point, and you figure, "What the heck? (Or "hell," "for shame!" or some other fancy moniker.) But you keep reading. Here are the words you see:

Age and illness will get in the way every time, but that shouldn't stop us. I may have mentioned this in other parts of this book, but will do so again here, I am in constant severe pain due to the operation I had on my leg in 2012, and there is no medicine that will relieve it, but I refuse to let that stop me from accomplishing my goals or living a happy life.

Rabbi Avi Taff of The Harold M. Schulweis Day School in Encino, California once said something in a speech that raised some important issues. His eloquent words, while not overly religious in context, spoke wonderfully to some of the themes of this book:

"America has afforded the individual the opportunity to make choices, and the question is: How do we as individuals approach life?"

From *The Station* by the poet and Reverend Robert J. Hastings:

"Tucked away in our subconscious is an idyllic vision. We see ourselves on a long trip that spans the continent. We are traveling by train. Out the windows we drink in the passing scene of cars on nearby highways, of children waving at a crossing, of cattle grazing on a distant hillside, of smoke pouring from a power plant, of row upon row of corn and wheat, of flatlands and valleys, of mountains and rolling hillsides, of city skylines and village halls. But uppermost in our minds is the final destination. Bands will be playing and flags waving. Once we get there our dreams will come true, and the pieces of our lives will fit together like a jigsaw puzzle. How relentlessly we pace the aisles, damming the minutes for loitering-waiting, waiting, waiting for the station."

And so, to the teen who is dreaming of reading this book, ask yourself the following (as *The Station* continues):

"When we reach the station, will that be it?
Will I cry?
When I'm eighteen?
When I buy a new 450sl Mercedes-Benz?
When I put the last kid through college?
When I have paid off the mortgage?
When I get a promotion?
When I reach the age of retirement?"

"Err ...what?" you may ask.

And I say to you:

Stop pacing the aisles and counting the miles! Instead, climb more mountains, eat more ice cream, go barefoot more often, swim more rivers, watch more sunsets, laugh more, and cry less. Life must be lived as we go along. The station will come soon enough.

Yes, we are born and we will die. Choosing life will enable us to arrive at our final destination knowing that we have arrived at peace with ourselves, healed of whatever evil we may have committed knowingly or unknowingly, and have hopefully left behind a better world than the one we traveled in.

In the final analysis, judging how successful the journey was can only be determined after it is completed.

So, you may have some time yet. But the time is now to start planning. Remember, enjoy your years. The way it works is this:

"Forty is the old age of youth; fifty is the youth of old age."

—Victor Hugo

SENIOR MOMENT #11

LIFE IS A CHALLENGE WORTH PURSUING

When you turn my age, we've established you may very well still feel like a kid in your mind, but not in your body, and in your spirit, but nowhere else.

It goes so ridiculously fast. It really does. And things do become blurred.

Kids, college, illness, dying...it ain't all fun, but it's realistic and needs to be seen as such.

The rest of this time will be written as a blur, as is life. Hopefully, you can capture some worthwhile nuggets of information in the pages that follow.

Here goes.

Ten…nine...eight…seven…six…five…four…three…two…one… Blast off!

Bernard Otis and His Wisdom Nuggets

(Or, Why This Outspoken Eighty-Five Year Old Believes He Has Earned the Right to Write This Book and Educate Each and Every One of You!)

I recently attended the 101st birthday party of my friend Marvin. He moves with a walker, has difficulty seeing and hearing, and yet he is always the life of the party. Marvin plays poker, as well as other games, with a group of older men once a week and usually comes away a winner. He could easily have given up on life many years ago, but he is determined to enjoy it until his time comes.

As a youngster growing up in Detroit, Michigan, I was always excited to read the poetry of Edgar A. Guest, a writer for a major newspaper. The following poem is one of my favorites, and I often carry it with me:

They Said It Couldn't Be Done

Somebody said it couldn't be done,
But he with a chuckle replied
That maybe it couldn't, but he would be one
Who wouldn't say, "Til he tried."

So he buckled right in with the trace of a grin
On his face. If he worried he hid it,
He started to sing as he tackled the thing
That couldn't be done, and he did it.

Somebody scoffed: "Oh, you'll never do that:
At least no one ever has done it."
But he took off his coat and he took off his hat
And the first thing he knew he'd begun it.

With the lift of his chin and a bit of a grin,
Without any doubting or quitting
He started to sing as he tackled the thing
That couldn't be done, and he did it.

There are thousands to tell you it cannot be done,
There are thousands to prophesy failure:
There are thousands to point out to you, one by one,

The dangers that wait to assail you,
But just buckle right in with a bit of a grin
Then take off your coat and go to it:
Just start in to sing as you tackle the thing
That cannot be done, and you'll do it.

While there may not be scientifically tested proof that keeping the mind active and involved adds years to a life, there certainly is a multitude of anecdotal evidence that by remaining involved in life, using our knowledge, talent, and even trying new things, we will certainly be happier as we move through our final years.

One of the most interesting things that came out of my research on this subject was that many persons I spoke with, young and aging, told me that they had a physical problem which they believed prevented them from doing something, and so they did not try.

They became so conditioned to avoiding any kind of physical activity because of that belief, but every once in a while one of them would attempt to perform the activity, such as walking a short distance, using a supposedly injured hand to paint, to do some other artistic work, and they were able to do it. When we condition our minds to believe we can't do something, we are restricting our ability to enjoy life.

In the September 23, 2013 issue of *Time* (how ironic), Jeffery Kluger wrote a most interesting article entitled, "The Art of Living." In it, he informs us that the *Medical Journal* reported a survey of 68,000 subjects in England which found that people with even relatively mild depression have a twenty-nine percent increased risk of dying from cardiovascular disease and a twenty-nine percent increased risk of dying from other non-cancerous disorders.

In the same article, Dr. George Bartzokis, a neurologist and professor of psychiatry at UCLA, is quoted as saying, "How well your brain does affects how well your body does."

Finally, Kluger reports that "Just last month, a research review published in *BMC Public Health* found that doing volunteer work in places such as hospitals and soup kitchens that allow direct contact with the people you're helping may lower mortality rates by as much as twenty-two percent compared with those of non volunteers."

Food for thought.

An attractive middle-aged couple is having marital problems and decides to go to a marriage counselor. They walk into the doctor's office and sit down. The doctor enters the room and begins to ask them a question and the wife goes ballistic and starts hollering and screaming. The doctor gets up and walks over to her and puts his arms around her as he gives her a very passionate kiss.

He then walks back to his chair and says to the husband, "Your wife needs that three times a week. The husband replies, "Okay, I can have her here Mondays, Wednesdays, and Fridays at three o'clock p.m.

SENIOR MOMENT #12

NO MATTER YOUR AGE, LIFE ENDS
WHEN YOU STOP LIVING IT

No, we're not there yet, so don't get nervous.

But, to answer: It ends when you stop living.

> "Once you have lost your curiosity about life, your sense
> of exploration, you have lost the gift of living."

> —James C. Humes

In his book, *Stories for Speakers,* Dr. Morris Mandel tells the story about an interview that John Dewey, the great philosopher, gave to a reporter shortly before Dewey's ninetieth birthday.

> "What is the good of all your thinking?" the
> reporter asked. "Where does it get you?"

> Dewey replied quietly, "The good is that
> which lies in climbing mountains."

> "Climbing mountains?" questioned the reporter.
> "What is the good of doing that?"

> "You see the other mountains," was the reply, followed by:
> "When you are no longer interested in climbing mountains
> to see other mountains to climb, then life is over."

Far too many people as they age and approach the end of their life close their eyes to life and do not see that each day brings new challenges, new adventures and new opportunities for living a happy and useful life. We see this in homes for the aged, in Assisted Living Centers and other similar situations.

For many years I have had the privilege, as a volunteer caregiver, to work with persons of all ages who either as a result of birth defect, illness, accidents or aging, have found themselves facing death.

Those who saw life as a challenge and lived each day looking forward to the next with excitement were the happiest and lived the longest. They sought new adventures, tried new activities, and wanted only, as the Author Letty Cottin Pogrebin noted during a recent book signing in Los Angeles, to be "treated with normalcy." They did not fear death and were excited about living each day in joy, despite their physical or mental impairments.

"Eternity does not happen after life, but every day of life."

—Rabbi Edward Feinstein
Valley Beth Shalom, Encino, C

The famous logo therapist, Victor E. Frankl, who believes that our primary drive in life is not pleasure, but the discovery of what we personally find meaningful, wrote in his Book, *Man's Search for Meaning*, "Man does not simply exist but always determines what his existence will be, what he will become in the next moment."

Frankl raises a good point. Basically, how can one be optimistic in light of the fact that life is filled with tragedy, challenges, illness, uncertainties, and death?

The answer of course, as Frankl wisely points out, is that we have to search for a reason to be happy just as we must find a reason to laugh. Yes, life is a challenge, but human beings are also given the inner strength to meet that challenge and live a life that is meaningful.

Usually when a writer undertakes a project such as this book, they spend many hours doing research and interviewing persons with experience in the subject matter they are writing about. And while I admit to having done that, it is also my good fortune to be blessed with close family members who have and are living the experience and who have each, in their own way, demonstrated that no matter what health, physical, or other burdens they must deal with, remaining active both physically and mentally, as well as committing oneself to living life to its fullest everyday, gives them much joy.

The following are two examples of that:

My cousin Bessie lived into her nineties, and despite all kinds of medical and physical problems, she lived life to its fullest almost until the day she died. She outlived two marriages by socializing, reading, shopping, and always looking for new adventures and new opportunities.

She refused to move to a care center even though she could hardly walk, and she insisted upon taking care of her own finances and other personal matters, much to the chagrin of her children, as well as those of us who spoke to her almost daily.

When she complained to me about having so much paperwork to do, I jokingly offered to do it for her if she would give me control of her money. We both got a laugh out of that.

Finally, one of the women I most admire is my cousin Jean Goldberg in Sherman Oaks, California. Now in her early eighties, Jean was challenged by a stroke while giving birth to her youngest daughter many years ago and has since spent most of her time in a wheelchair. She lives at home with a caregiver, looks wonderful, has a happy life and attitude, gets out, and is actively involved in living. It is impossible to leave a visit with her without having learned a lesson about how wonderful the travel through life can be—despite the obstacles.

These are just a few of the examples of persons who understand the value of the gift of life and making every minute count. When we stop using our minds and limit our physical and social activities, we have stopped living.

SENIOR MOMENT #13

RELATIONSHIPS ARE ONE OF OUR MOST VALUABLE ASSESTS

The most valuable of all things that add to our will to live are loving, social, and personal relationships. I see this time and time again among the elderly. When two people share their lives, they increase the quality of the their lives. Enter any senior long-term care facility and watch in amazement as those in their late years help each other and enjoy their time together.

Martin Buber in his *I and Thou* talks about the **I** and **It** versus the **I** and **You.** When we live alone and have no close friends, we are the **I** and all others are the **It**.

We have no relationship with those we come into contact with, but when we establish a relationship and get to know each other, and in a sense have a companionship, the **It** becomes **You,** and we are no longer alone.

Ask yourself, "How many times each day do we interact with persons we don't know and never make an attempt to form warm relationships which could add so much to the quality of our lives?"

I am reminded of a story that James C. Humes—an author, speaker, and speechwriter for Richard Nixon—tells in his *Speaker's Treasury of Anecdotes about the Famous,* a work that is source of many of the quotations included in the book you are now holding.

Once, when Daniel Webster ran into John Adams and asked how he was feeling, Adams drew a steep sigh and said, "I inhabit a weak, frail, decayed tenement, battered by the winds, and broken in upon the storms, and from what I can learn, the landlord does not intend to repair.

*(*Author's comment: Even though repairs will not be made, the lower level of the tenement can be made comfortable if the upper level remains active.)

A HUMOROUS STORY ABOUT JOHN AND SARAH

John was not feeling well, so Sarah took him to the doctor. Following the examination, while John was in the dressing room, the doctor called Sarah aside and said to her, "John is a good candidate for a stroke or heart attack, so here is what I want you to do: Each day when he returns from work, have him do absolutely nothing but rest. Give him a very good dinner, and at least three times a week have sexual relations with him." As the doctor left, John came out of the dressing room. He asked Sarah what the doctor had said. She replied, "He told me you are going to die."

Let me grow lovely, growing old
So many fine things do:
Laces, and ivory, and gold,
And silks may not be new.
And there is healing in old trees,
Old streets a glamour hold:
Why may not I, as well as these,
Grow lovely, growing old?

—Karl Wilson Baker

Life can end before death when you give up on it. It can end when you abandon the opportunity to use what capabilities you have to enjoy it, teach others, and wait for the end to naturally occur.

Ruth and Burt are a remarkably wonderful couple with a large, warm family. They are in their late eighties and have been married approximately eighteen years.

He has a number of health issues and is unable to walk well so he uses an electric cart. His neuropathy gives him great pain, but despite this, they are happily in love. She does her very best to make certain he is as comfortable as possible even though she also has aging problems, and while some days are very difficult for both of them, they are most happy, fun to be with couple. They prove every day that life can be joyful and are the perfect example of those who choose life.

SENIOR MOMENT #14

OUR FAMILY'S IMPORTANCE AS WE AGE
I AM MY BROTHER'S KEEPER

"The Lord said to Cain, "Where is your brother Abel?"
And Cain replied, "I do not know. Am I my brother's keeper?"

—Genesis 4.9

Are we our brothers' keeper? This is a question that has, throughout the history of mankind, begged for an answer. As Rabbi Sheldon Zimmerman has pointed out in *The Modern Men's Torah Commentary*, it is the first question directed to God in the Torah.

But let's say you're not religious. No matter. Let's talk about family.

When you get right down to it, there is no element more essential in the process of living and dying than the need to have good family relationships.

But again, let's take a converse view: Let's say you are married with no children. You may have a dog; you may have a cat. You may even have a parakeet.

It's all family.

Unless the matters discussed in this chapter are properly addressed early on, all of the other information presented in this book regarding resources and life's meaning will be of little help in resolving the main issues of aging.

Challenges are a part of life, but needless challenges should never be acceptable. We have the power both individually and collectively to take actions that will minimize it and move on with enjoying the time we are given.

Yes, families have their differences, jealousies, and misunderstandings. If you really think about it, some of the issues that divide us are, in reality, petty. Nevertheless, we are all brothers and sisters, and if we follow our hearts we are responsible for one another.

While it is not possible to know when we will suddenly find ourselves or a family member being struck with such diseases as Parkinson's, Dementia, Alzheimer's, or any other long-term condition, the affect that it has is devastating to not only to the challenged, but also the spouse who potentially becomes a full-time caregiver. A full-time caregiver, whether at home or in a care center, can potentially end the love relationship and replace it with loneliness and emotional stress.

When the joy of marriages which have lasted many years come to an end because of the death of one of the partners or due to a serious illness such as Alzheimer's, the other spouse now finds themselves under the mental and physical strain of dealing with health, financial, and other losses which seem to appear from nowhere.

> "Be nice to your children. After all, they will be
> the one's choosing your nursing home."
>
> —Anonymous

In order to avoid, or at the least minimize, these kinds of stressful situations, there are a number of actions that need to be taken early in a marriage. This is not only because they make for a happier life for all concerned, but also because they serve to build the foundation for the aging needs of our elderly loved ones and our own as well.

The family must take into consideration early the possible deterioration of the sick person's health, either as result of the strain of dealing with their partner's issues or their own aging process.

Consider this: Recent studies by the Center for Disease Control and many other reputable sources indicate that the spouse of a person who dies as a result of a major disease often dies within a short time after the of the death of their family member. Everything needs to be discussed with legal representation and properly documented so as to avoid problems if, or when, the need to implement them arises.

In 1991, Anna and I returned from a trip to England where we have many friends. We called to check our phone messages and learned that her eighty-three-year-old father had been challenged by a stroke that day. Tired and exhausted, we drove 130 miles to the hospital where he stayed and began the many months of the costly vigil that ended in his death.

At the same time, as we were draining our resources for his care, we learned that Anna's youngest sister at forty-two years old had incurable breast cancer. She was twice divorced and had two sons: a nineteen year old and a twelve year old.

Because they lived a short distance from us we did know the boys well, but when we were told at the City of Hope that the sister only had a short time to live, Anna and I immediately agreed that we would adopt the youngest boy—which we did. It turned out to be disaster and eventually we had to make other arrangements for him.

The reasons are not important here save for one:

These two events, along with several other family tragedies, literally wiped us out financially. However, we continued our careers and eventually overcame those problems. We believed then, as I do now, that we are all our brothers' keepers—meaning we all need to take care of our own.

It should be obvious to anyone reading about these costly events that had the family discussed and planned for these kinds of issues—the illness and death of an aging man, as well as the sudden illness and death of a single mother with children—the financial drain endured might have been minimized.

Each person in life is given a choice to live with goodness or evil. When we put the puzzle pieces on a table and try to put it together, it is hard to understand, but if we look at the picture on the box it came in, we can better understand how to put the pieces together.

Sadly, there are situations which happen over the years that put a family member into a position where they honestly believe that in order to save their family, they have to act in a manner that is contrary to what they believe. They end up doing harm to themselves, losing the respect of those they love, and being challenged by a lifetime of inner pain just to protect another family member.

Sadly, that is their choice and their burden to carry.

Divided families need to look at themselves as the picture on the cover of puzzle box and learn how to reassemble the pieces so that they are there for each other in times of need.

It is mind-boggling to me to see how really foolish some of the issues are and that in the whole of the scheme of life, families allow themselves to become split apart.

Some of the greatest polarizers in split families are the following:

Religious Differences

If religion, most of which teach us to love one another, helps others when times are difficult and encourage us to multiply and grow, then how can it possibly be so acrimonious?

I know, I know. This is a very large question, in some ways well out of the scope of this book. But let me try to get to the heart of the matter anyway.

I recently learned of a family whose daughter married a very religious man. Because the parents were not as religious, they were not allowed to visit or eat in the daughter's home. Sadly, the daughter died from cancer in her fifties, and not until her final days were her loving parents allowed to spend time with her.

This is a typical issue, unfortunately. Here's another, though, that's more accepting. This one proves it can all work:

I met a family where the husband was of one faith and the wife of another. They had been married for close to thirty-five years and were very much in love. Their children were raised in their mother's faith but were fully knowledgeable about their father's religious upbringing. The family celebrated holidays of both faiths as well.

Due to successful family dynamics like this, I could never understand why family relationships should be ruined over these kinds of issues. My aunt and uncle were of different political beliefs, but they were also happily married for over fifty years.

My conclusion: Live and let live. People are different by nature. You can't expect them all to be clones, can you?

Racial Issues

The daughter of a very happy family fell in love and eventually married a man of a different race than hers. She knew of her father's prejudice and hid the relationship from him. When it finally became publicly known, the father refused to have a relationship with his daughter or her wonderful husband.

See "Religious Differences" above. It's the same damn thing.

Giving Birth "Out of Wedlock"

This is a generational thing. People don't even talk like this anymore.

But, for this purpose, let's talk about it anyway. When a young woman becomes pregnant "out of wedlock," whether from a loving relationship or a casual one, families have difficulty dealing with it. All too often, they disown the child at a time when the need is for their parents, family, and friends to put their arms around them and give them love.

Again—as I'm well into my eighties—I need to acknowledge that even listing this one here may reek of "old fashioned" nonsense. But it's my book, and it'll reek if I want it to!

So…a client of mine told me that his young daughter was pregnant and was moving across the country to live with a cousin. I asked him why, and he told me that neither he nor his wife wanted anything to do with her because of the "out of wedlock" child.

I told him he was wrong and that he needed to embrace his daughter and give her love. Due to my wife Anna's illness, I did not see him again for close to a year. When I asked him if he had heard from his daughter and how she and her child were doing, he told me that he had taken my advice and that they were all living together. He said they could not be happier.

Divorce and Custody Issues

There is the story of a very successful young woman who had a very unhappy marriage. She divorced her husband and, in the process, both she and her in-laws (and other family members) stopped seeing and speaking to each other. She is raising the son born into the marriage and he is a delightful young man, now in his preteens, who is very actively involved in community work.

The mother is devoted to her son and has maintained her successful career. After many years of separation, the in-laws contacted her to speak about reconciliation. She is absolutely thrilled and happily looking forward to her son finally getting to know his paternal grandparents and family. That is what life should be about.

Family. Always, family.

Another example of the necessity of a familial support system is after a long and usually happy marriage, the spouses wake up one day and find that due to a sudden illness, aging problem, or the death of their mate, their life has disintegrated and their very survival—financially or otherwise—has become an unbearable ordeal.

What better way to minimize this kind of problem than for every member of a family to work together, love together, and plan together early in the journey. That way, when such a situation arises, they are prepared to deal with it.

Yes, all of us—me included—have, at times, had serious disagreements or ill feelings with other members of our family and/or done some things that affected our family relationships. But when you really think about it, what can be so terrible as to cause us to sever and throw cold water on those relationships and not be there for each other in times of crisis?

Nothing. Nothing at all.

I was going to end this chapter here, and then I just heard about this story on the radio:

A family has several children and grandchildren. One daughter has a young son with a physical disability. They have not spoken for years, and now the boy is dying. He was interviewed on the radio begging for the return of his family before he arrived in Heaven.

How terribly sad.

SENIOR MOMENT #15

DO NOT STORE YOUR AGING LOVED ONES AWAY

"We Interrupt This Program for a Special Report"

I am writing this on Sunday, July 14, 2013. I am watching CNN on the television.

They are reporting that the Chinese government has just passed a new law. This new law is requiring the families of aging persons living in care centers to be required to visit their loved ones at least once every two months.

They are actually announcing this as if it's a special report.

This is so interesting to me, and yet also so sad to think that a law has to be passed requiring families to help one another, no matter the reason they stopped.

These words follow along with the last chapter, but I placed them here, separately, as my mind is blown. Is this what we've come to as a society?

———◆———

Unfortunately, all too often as our loved ones age and our society becomes more mobile, the distances between us physically and mentally leave the elderly alone and sad.

For my younger readers, this is a true-blue, honest issue. When you are old enough to feel this pain, you will understand. For now, please try to understand; it's all I can ask.

The fact is that many families use care centers as "babysitters" as they wait for their sick family member to die, while they go about enjoying life on the money that the family has accumulated. One needs only to spend time in any care center to see this phenomenon in action.

There is a subtle change taking place in our society that is slowly and significantly affecting the needs of the aging. Almost all persons involved in the care of the elderly realize that:

1. Many of the elderly under their care have no children, and thus must rely almost entirely on close family or friends to care for them.

2. A large portion of the elderly patients has never married or is divorced. This again makes them more dependent on others.

3. The cost of entering a care facility is increasing at a rapid rate and makes it less possible for many to be able to afford to be there. Being wiped out financially is a common result.

The quality of life for an aging person depends as much on their relationship with loved ones as it does on their actual physical condition. What aging persons want more than anything else is the feeling of normalcy, knowing that they still play an integral part in and are still part of their family's activities.

If they have no biological family, then we can insert the word "friends" in its place. If they have no friend, well, perhaps you didn't listen to Grandpa Bernie and *plan*.

Companionship in any form helps an elderly person keep their mind as vibrant as possible as their journey continues. Yes, it may be difficult to take them outside, take them away from their normal life, and take the time to care for them, but most of our aged loved ones have devoted their lives to us and had many of the same time constraints. Now, it is our turn to reciprocate.

The parent becomes the child, and the child becomes the parent.

In the early 2000s I had volunteered to head up the Bikkur Holim Program (caring for the sick) at my Synagogue. My close friend and respected Rabbi, Edward Feinstein at Valley Beth Shalom in Encino, California, called and asked me to see if I could assist the family of one of his friends who had Lou Gehrig's disease.

Gary was a very well-known professional who had two grown sons. He was divorced and lived on his own with a caregiver. He was mostly in a wheelchair and always tube-fed; he could no longer speak and communicated via a computer program.

His family and I met and discussed his condition and needs which were helping him in having some sort of normalcy during his journey to the end. Due to this meet up, he and I began a one-and-a-half year, heartwarming relationship.

I had made a new friend. A kind, loving new friend.

As it turned out, Gary had been the camp counselor at the summer camp my children had attended many years prior to our meeting.

Every Wednesday, Gary and I would spend three hours together, during which time we discussed his feelings about life and death, played various card games, and discussed family relationships. I arranged with the Braille Institute to have books on tape sent to him.

Additionally, Anna, who among her many professional talents was a teacher of Meditation, visited him once a week and taught Gary how to use Meditation as a way of easing his pain.

There were three issues of concern to all of us. First, while the family wanted to take him out on occasion, Gary felt uncomfortable being seen in his condition. Second, one of his family members was about to get married in a few months and again he was reluctant to attend the event. Finally, the religious holidays were approaching and he did not want to go to the services.

We addressed all of these matters, and slowly Gary realized that not only did he have needs, which his family had addressed by bringing our religious leaders into the process, but that they also had the need to share their love and commitment to him by involving him in the family events.

Through careful planning of transportation, aides, seating, and special entry into the various facilities involved, he did join in the various family events moving forward.

Reluctantly, he agreed to attend his son's wedding. On the day after, with tears in his eyes, he told me that is was one of the most meaningful days of his life. In fact, on the day we took him to services for the Jewish New Year, there was not a dry eye in the Synagogue as he sat proudly with his family gathered around him.

Unfortunately, Gary passed away the day after I had emergency heart surgery. I felt as though I lost a brother. Anna attended his services and reported how warm they were and how satisfied the family was that his journey had a happy ending.

Gary, my friend, Bernie misses you tremendously. I can only hope I helped you decrease that gulf of distance you felt in your heart for so long.

> "The human brain is like a tarnished piece of gold that sits in a cabinet.
> You cannot keep it shined and bright unless you use it regularly.
> So think before you act, and treat others as they treat you!"

—Guess who? Me.

If I had to point to one issue that was more difficult for all parties—those who were seriously ill, as well as the families and friends of those who had passed on—it is the "trauma" so many have with having to visit with them or pay their respects.

Time and again during my research, individuals told me how angry they were with the fact that persons who they considered close friends had failed to call, visit, or acknowledge or show concern in any way their loss.

Just as there is a tendency to avoid speaking about death, when it's time to make a decision about visiting the sick, attending funerals, and visiting mourners, a large proportion of humankind fears having to get involved or to reach out to those who are in need. And, many who know they should do so have guilt feelings and avoid acting because they are afraid that they may do or say the wrong thing.

We all, at one time or another, have had this kind of experience. There are tons of stories about how close friendships and otherwise wonderful relationships have been affected both positively and negatively by the manner in which individuals handle this situation.

Similarly, many who are also going through the pain and challenges do not want to speak about their ordeal and/or are sometimes upset with their friends' reactions.

All those who have been caretakers through volunteering, in their personal lives, and millions of individuals who have dealt with this issue through their and their family's own struggle with illness and aging all pretty much agree that there are three basic beliefs we all share about what people in such situations want when it comes to interaction:

1. Our Privacy

Nobody, least of all a person who is seriously ill, wants his or her situation broadcasted to the world. Of course it is important for us to know that family, friends and acquaintances are concerned about us, but they need to show their concerns in ways that will not disturb our privacy.

Any calls, personal notes, and, if appropriate, brief personal contact, from our family members just to let us know that your thoughts are with us, are okay.

2. Normalcy

One the most important things that a sick person wants is "normalcy."

No matter where we are in life, we want to know that we are not alone and that we are involved in life and that of the world around us. It is most important that our loved ones, as well as our caregivers, keep this in mind when working to help us through our varied illnesses and crises.

3. Focus. And the focus needs to be on "them," not "us."

When speaking with or visiting a sick person, do not talk about your experiences with an illness, or that of others (as in people you know who may have had a similar health problem).

Listen to what the person(s) you are with are relating to you about their situation and keep quiet. Put your hand gently on their shoulder or hold their hand and listen carefully.

If you, as a loved one of the sick person, are asked by a friend if they can visit that person and you give your permission, be certain to tell them that during their visit they must concentrate on the person they are visiting and not talk about themselves or their experiences. Be sure to tell them how long they can stay.

Irene Winston is one of the most dynamic women I have ever met. She is in her nineties, cannot walk on her own, and has more ailments than you can shake a stick at. She has also, until recently, had a group of women friends who come to the facility where she lives twice a week, where they played the usual card games with her.

In addition, Irene attended a weekly political discussion with a group of others in the facility. Her family knows better than to do anything to keep this wonderfully warm human "out of the loop of life."

Irene recently took a bad fall and has been moved to a new care center. I visited her and found her as mentally alert as one could expect at her age, and as feisty as ever. Although she cannot walk and needs more assistance, she remains *in life*.

Sadly, Irene would be challenged by a stroke shortly before the completion of this book, and just a day or so after visiting with her entire family and sharing memories and words of love with them, she passed away at the age of ninety-five. Following the eulogies of one of the most beautiful services I have ever attended, the guitarists played and sang "Goodnight Irene." What a great way to say goodbye.

Another related story: A prominent and community-oriented family (I have chosen not to identify them publicly) had a daughter who for many years had to live in a well-known medical facility because of a genetic disease. (The family actually was among the founders of a national foundation which supports the research for that illness.)

Upon graduation from a high school at the medical center, the daughter was returning home to arrange to attend a major college when she was killed in an automobile accident.

I had to travel a distance to get to the funeral and arrived late, but I was able to get to the parents' home following the services. I put my arms around the girls and the mother and said, "Nobody can feel your pain, but I have nothing but empathy for you and the family."

The mother began to cry, hugged me back and said, "Of all of those who are here today, you are the first person who understands."

This experience is not here to enhance my image, but rather to demonstrate how important it is to keep your eye on the bouncing ball when in such situations.

Let me also stress that while we may think that we need to shield our children from the subject of life's dark side, our young children also have feelings, and they see and hear what's going on in our lives. It is so much better for us, as well as them, to be open and, in a calm and positive atmosphere, discuss these issues with them.

The following story, better that anything I can write, exemplifies this. After you have digested it and wiped the tears from your eyes, I will identify those involved:

There was a man who was visiting some friends for a holiday dinner. His wife lay near death in a hospital. His hosts were being visited by two of their grandchildren from out of state—a boy, eleven, and a girl, ten. Prior to the man's arrival, the host had informed them of their guest's situation.

As dessert was being served, the man excused himself and said that he needed to leave early so that he could go by the hospital and kiss his wife goodnight. She died later that evening, and the hosts informed his grandchildren the next morning.

Two weeks later, the man called his host and asked if he was sitting down. He said no, and the man said please sit down, as I want to read something to you.

He then read a note that he had received from the granddaughter of his host. In the letter, she expressed her deep sadness over the death of the man's wife, promised him her love and support, and told him that he should gather strength from the fact that, as her mom had told her, the man's wife was now with God. In closing, she said that should the man needed anything he should, please call her and let her know.

Two grown men were bawling their eyes out during that conversation.

The host then called the young girl's mother to see if she knew about the note that her daughter had sent. She was completely and, of course, pleasantly surprised, although her daughter had already told her about the death.

Two weeks later the child wrote the following note to the man as a follow up to his note of gratitude to her:

Dear _____,

I was really excited to finally hear from you. It was especially happy to hear that writing your new book helped with some of your grief. I know I told you this before, but anytime you want to write to get more grief away, I'm always here.

Me and my mom talked about it a lot, and my mom told me that dying is a happy thing because you are then reunited with God. I hope you are feeling better because I know from what you told me in your letter to me that you had gotten a lot of letters. Well, I have to go. Hope to hear from you soon. My brother Ryan says to tell you "hi" and is also very sorry for your loss.

Best wishes always.

These words of wisdom from the mind of my then ten-year-old granddaughter, Jennifer, came unsolicited to my dear fried rabbi Edward Zerin, whose tragic story I told earlier in this book.

How could there be any greater example of the reason why such matters have such an effect on every person, and why young and old alike need to openly share life's happiness and sadness?

"Mitzvah" is a Jewish term for doing good. There is no better way to describe how beneficial it is to reach out and demonstrate your love for someone close than to do a "Mitzvah" for them when they are going through life threatening situations...but it is also critical that you do so in a way that makes the sick person feel safe and comfortable.

In addition to the three suggestions I discussed earlier in this chapter, the following are a number of additional guidelines that most professional caregivers agree can help your efforts be successful:

1. Informing your close ones that you have a problem.

    Certainly, when a person first learns that they have a serious or potentially serious health problem, it is shocking, mentally draining, and instills them with fear.

    And while immediate family members obviously need to be informed, others who are close need to step back and give their primary parties a chance to collect their thoughts, get their medical diagnosis in order, and establish a strategy for dealing with the situation.

    By leaving a message on your phone, as well as an "out of office" type message on your email informing callers that you appreciate their call and concern, you will have taken the first step towards keeping everyone calm. Inform them through these messages that you have an illness, need time to deal with its treatment, and will notify them when you and/or your family will be available with more information. Sign off by expressing love for the caller.

    If, as in many situations, the number of phone messages is overwhelming, leave an appropriate message indicating how the caller can obtain information, or have another person handle the responses. You can also leave a recorded message updating the information on daily basis, or every few days.

2. Try to eliminate the question "how are you?" from your vocabulary.

Whether it is in a business or personal contact with others, these three words are the most useless and wasted in the dictionary. No one really cares how anyone is. What we want to know is what are they thinking? What are they doing? What are their concerns? Think about this for a moment: You ask me, "How are you?" I say, "I am terrible," "I don't feel well," or "I have a cold." Now tell me what can you possible say that will alleviate my feelings or give you incentive to carry on that conversation?

3. Call the sick person or a family member and make sure a visit is okay and, if so, when would be the best time.

Also ask what you can do to help them, or what you can bring to them that would be beneficial. Be very careful about bringing flowers. Many persons have allergies to them. Also, be sensitive to their situation and do not wear perfumes or other aroma-bearing toiletries.

Oftentimes the person you are visiting may be too embarrassed to ask you to leave. Use good sense and do not overstay your visit.

4. Have a clear purpose for your visit.

Always keep in mind that the person you are visiting is dealing with a serious health problem. They generally do not want small talk. You are there to comfort them and show how much you care for them.

5. What to do if others are present?

Avoid carrying on conversations quietly or in another room—where the sick person can overhear you—with others who may be there during your visit. I did this inadvertently during Anna's illness and she was most upset. Rightfully so.

6. Do not ask about medical equipment and other devices you see.

No matter what personal property or medical devices you observe during your visit, do not ask about them.

7. Where to sit during your visit

Unless there is no alternative, do not stand next to the patient during your visit. Be aware of any hearing problem they have so that you can modulate your voice accordingly.

8. What to talk about

   As suggested earlier, let the patient lead the conversation. While it is okay in most cases to inquire about their situation, do so in a non-aggressive manner and do not push them about it.

   During your visit—particularly if it is in a hospital or some care facility—there may very well be interruptions during your visit for medical/nursing attention, so choose you words carefully and with some intent, such as offering to assist the sick person, or their family, with tasks they have to accomplish, household chores, etc.

9. What to say when greeting mourners at funerals and in their homes

   Whether attending the funeral or visiting the family of a person we knew and cared for—or that of a member of the family of someone we know—the degree of sadness that permeates the scene depends upon the age of the deceased and the cause of death.

   Again, it is important to express your sad feelings without being dramatic. For example, do not say, "I know how you feel," "She was so young at heart," or "Life can be so unfair." Sometimes just hugging the bereaved sends the right message.

   As I have, in an earlier example, explained that no one but the person you are visiting can feel his or her pain. Don't try.

   All too often, friendships and lost families are broken up, and sadness is added to those who are ill or in mourning because friends say the wrong thing and try to equate themselves with the one who is grieving. Better to say nothing or simply hug or touch the person and convey your grief silently. They know why you are there.

"Sometimes our physical presence is enough to comfort or encourage others. I am reminded of the little girl who went to comfort the mother of a classmate who had recently died. When she returned home, the little girl's mother asked her what she had done to comfort her friend's mother. The little girl softly replied, 'I just sat on her lap and cried with her.'"

—Glenn Van Ekeren, *The Speaker's Sourcebook*

At Anna's funeral—both in the chapel and at the gravesite—while we had a most moving religious service, I told everyone in attendance that I wanted them to leave the grounds that day in a happy and celebrative frame of mind. I wanted them all to be forever grateful that we had had this magnificent woman in our lives for so many years. To my way of thinking, a celebration of life is the best way to honor a lost loved one.

10. Dealing with sadness and tears.

While we should always be upbeat and positive when visiting the sick or mourners—not to say we should be full of laughs and be telling funny stories—there certainly are times when that just is not possible and we should do our best not to let the sadness overwhelm us.

Earlier this year, a man who I had grown up and been friends with for seventy-nine years lay near death in a local hospital. Because his wife had difficulty driving I took her to visit him and spent about an hour with him.

His mind had deteriorated and he was very confused, but he did know me and we were able to communicate our feelings. As I left the room, we both knew that it would be the last time we would see each other, and he began to sob. Naturally, I could not hold back, and as we said our goodbyes I broke down and left the room.

Express your sorrow over their loss. Tell them you have deep empathy for them. Let them know how much you admired their lost loved one, recall happy stories about them.

—❖—

"Life is the spin we put on it. We cannot control everything that happens
to us. However, the meaning we give to what happens is within our
control. We can choose to cry at life, and we can choose to laugh.
We can waste our lives, or we can make our lives worthwhile.

That does not mean that everything will be perfect, nor that
we will get everything we want, or even that we necessarily
must take everything that comes our way. What it does mean
is that whatever our lot, we can make the most of it."

—Rabbi Edward Zerin, PH.D.
A Prisoner of Love

Edward is my close friend, a learned Rabbi, writer, and teacher. He's still active and doing
his thing in his mid nineties! God bless him.

SENIOR MOMENT #16

ALWAYS HELP OTHERS CREATE HAPPY PATHS

"We put more effort into helping folks reach old
age than into helping them enjoy it."

—Frank A. Clark

As a result of my work in the community, I have met some truly wonderful people who, for all of the reasons that are mentioned throughout the book, have found it necessary to move out of their homes and live in various types of care centers.

Many of them have families who live at a distance who do not visit as often as they should.

At a minimum, just a phone call every day can make a huge difference in the happiness of a loved one, and it makes them feel connected. The opposite effect happens when there is no such connection between the family members.

Good people make that call. Be good, people, because that's what you really are.

"Caring is the art of sharing. If you want to lift
yourself up, lift up someone else."

—Booker T. Washington

My longtime friend, Laurie Caplan-Shern, is a life coach and another one of the "good ones." I met her along with her husband, Steven, while on a cross-country plane ride. Laurie had written her own remarkable book abut the aging process, *Giving Birth to My Parents,* in which she describes how she realized that the life of her parents had begun to change as they aged. She discussed how important it was for her to heal the wounds of a sometimes rocky relationship with them. This way, they would enjoy being a close family for once, a process which helped her parents' journey to the end.

Laurie also told me what happiness that reconciliation brought to her own life.

My friend and spiritual leader, Rabbi Edward Feinstein, once relayed to his congregation the story of a special store he once visited. This store was in San Francisco where it sold beautiful ceramics. He noticed a "magnificent ceramic box made of dozens of colorful fragments," as he explained to me later, "a sort of three dimensional collage" that he was possibly interested in purchasing.

He asked the storeowner what it was. He was told that in China they have many earthquakes, after which the families gather up the large pieces of broken shards and they take them to a craftsman who creates a uniquely beautiful artifact from them.

This is the piece he was interested in.

Rabbi Feinstein relates this to the observance of the Jewish Day of Atonement, Yom Kippur, during which Jews come together every year to start anew and disavow the wrongs of the past year (as do other religions during their various religious practices). These wrongs usually related to "struggling with life, struggling to do the right thing, and struggling to say the right thing."

"What better way, then," Feinstein asks, "to renew ourselves than to be present for one another, to help one another, and gather all the broken pieces—the broken promises, the plans that failed to come about, the intentions never realized, the hopes that never came to be. In other words, to gather all of the shards of the past and put them together into beautiful relationships that will enrich our lives, as well as those of our loved ones as the journey through the years nears its destination."

Beautiful words.

So...

After that, I'm reminded of a Jewish-themed joke. Don't shoot; I'm just the messenger.

> Sarah was the last of the young women in her family to get married. She was a quite simple woman who came from a small family, and it took some time for her to meet the right man.

> On the Saturday morning after the wedding, all of her friends gathered at the synagogue, anxious to find out how she was enjoying her new

married life. They waited and waited, and just as the services were about to end, Sarah arrived looking exhausted and bedraggled.

"So Sarah," they asked, "how is married life?"

"Well," she said in a soft voice with a slight smile, "it's good."

"And your husband," they asked, "is he a good man?"

Sarah replied, "Last night was our first Sabbath Dinner as husband and wife. So I prepared a lovely meal just like my momma had taught me, and I set up a lovely table.

My husband came to the table and was very impressed. I lit the Sabbath Candles and recited the blessings. My husband then said to me, 'Sarah, it was the custom in my grandfather's home that after the lighting of the Sabbath Candles, he would take my grandmother upstairs to be together as husband and wife.' So upstairs we went.

An hour or so later, we came down and sat at the table and my husband raised the wine cup and recited the blessing. Then he said, 'Sarah, it was the custom in my uncle's home that after saying the blessing over the wine, my aunt and uncle went upstairs to be together as husband and wife.' So we went upstairs.

An hour or so later after that, we came down and sat at the table and he raised the Challah (egg bread) and said the blessing over the bread. Then he said, 'Sarah, it was the custom in my cousin's home that after saying the blessing over the bread, my cousin would take his wife upstairs to be together as husband and wife.' So we went upstairs. And this was repeated with the soup, the main meal, and desert.

So now you ask how married life is? And how is my husband? I'll tell you. Wealthy, he is not. Handsome, he is not. A scholar, he is not. But boy, does he have a wonderful family."

SENIOR MOMENT #17

COMPANIONSHIP AND LOVE ARE
NOT JUST FOR THE YOUNG

I recently came across some of the most beautiful and inspiring words written by the poet Merrit Malloy. They express, better than I can, the sentiments that Anna and I spoke to each other about during her final days. They also reflect on my own views that the death of a loving partner should not end the love affair, but rather take it to higher plains.

When I die
If you need to weep
Cry for someone
Walking the street beside you.

And when you need me
Put your arms around others
And give them what you need to give me.

You can love me most by letting
Hands touch hands, and
Souls touch souls.

You can love me most by
Sharing your joys
Multiplying your good deeds.

You can love me most by
Letting me live in your eyes
And not in your mind.

And when you say Kaddish (a prayer) for me
Remember that our Torah teaches,

Love doesn't die
People do.

So when all that's left of me is love
Give me away.

As this stage of life began to interest me more and more, I naturally began to think about my own situation and what my personal thoughts were. After all, I had a most remarkable thirty-year relationship with Anna, who had passed away just a few months prior to the start of this book.

One of the most difficult things for persons of age and in similar situations is to make others understand that we are not looking to be "fixed up" and that we do not have a "need." Rather, it is about "sharing," or a "want."

Companionship.

The last thing I was looking for when I moved into an assisted living center was companionship and romance. In fact, I was often kidded by friends who would ask me how I handled being with so many single women and I responded by saying that the thought never entered my mind—which it did not.

⊷❖⊷

Mary was close to sixty years of age and Joe was in his seventies. They had been married for thirty-five years. One night Joe said to Mary, "Do you realize that some thirty-five years ago, I had a low rent apartment, a small, compact car, I slept on my couch watched a small TV set, and whenever I wanted to, I could sleep with a sexy young blonde? Now I have a big home, a king-size bed, and the latest widescreen TV. I have a custom automobile, go out to the finest restaurants, travel the world and entertain at lavish parties in my home, and I am sleeping with a sixty-two-year-old blonde."

Mary thought about this for a moment and then responded by saying, "Sweetheart, you go out out and find a sexy young blonde and I will see to it that you once again have the low rent apartment, small car, a couch to sleep on, and a small TV."

Over the next few months, several things happened that caused me to take a hard look at my feelings about aging and romance, and I reflected upon the words of the poet William Butler Yeats:

> Wine comes in at the mouth
> And love comes in at the eyes:
> That's all we shall know for truth
> Before we grow old and die.

Since I am still mentally quite independent, I found living among a group of persons who were mostly more confined and many whose lives had, for the most part, slowed down because of both physical and memory issues, to be most challenging.

I did meet a few women with whom I had a social relationship. Not many. However, because at that time the one I most admired was not interested in a long-term involvement, it was the same for me as having nobody.

Unfortunately, as I got more involved in writing this book and also because rumors about my relationships got out of control, it became harder to maintain *any* relationships.

As I sadly discovered, when you live in a "closed environment," such as an assisted living center, you become suspect to being self-serving and no matter how sincere your intentions are, the other parties simply are not open to relationships and tend to question all you do.

It took me some time to realize that instead of trying to blend in, I needed to be myself. Thus, my life has once again reinvented—at eighty-four years old—and I continue to grow. I've made certain acceptances in my world and once again live a happy life. I make new friends, as well as enhance my existing long-time relationships outside of the environment where I live.

As I spoke about this to many single men and women my age, I learned that a few, but not many, also wanted companionship, but more so because they felt alone than for reasons of love.

What my "want" is to be with a person with whom I can share an emotional and loving connection; one who enjoys life and looks forward to every day with great anticipation, regardless of any physical restrictions they may have.

It would be my desire to respect her independence, encourage her to use her knowledge and creativity to, as best she could, help others and live a useful and productive life. And always enjoy cuddling in each other's arms.

While I do not share the commonly held view that older persons should not be companions or marry those younger than themselves for fear of death, that to me is absurd because no one knows what tomorrow will bring. Today, you can have so much joy regardless of age, if you allow it. If the motivation is sincere and not selfish than age differences do not seem to me to be an obstacle to happiness.

I recently met a woman in her seventies. She was visiting a nursing home and I interviewed her for this book. She told me that she was there to see her husband who had been confined for three years as a result of Alzheimer's and other health issues. She confided in me that after fifty-four years of marriage, he became very ill and her entire life had changed. While they had a happy marriage, taking care of him had drained her and there was no longer any love between them. She was lonely.

Eventually, she began a relationship with a widower and was open and upfront about it. She was very happy with their relationship. At the same time, she was committed to doing what she could to make her husband comfortable.

Healthcare professionals have told me that this situation is not unusual due to the added years medical science has given us. In fact, if anyone had told me that I would outlive a woman (Anna was twelve years my junior), I would have told him or her that they were not thinking clearly.

I do expect that, someday, the love that I shared with Anna will reside in the heart of another. And while this bothered me at first, I realized that it is simply unrealistic to believe that once you have had a magnificent love in your life that you can never have another.

> "Wisdom is the quality that keeps you from getting
> into situations where you need it."

—Doug Larsen

As I have mentioned previously, sometimes the good things we do for unselfish reasons are seen by others as self-serving. We need to take that into consideration as we move through life.

In an earlier chapter, I wrote about my relationship with Rabbi Ed Zerin and how the tragedy of his wife Marjory's accident brought us together. What I did not describe was how this remarkable man in his mid-nineties went on—despite some illnesses related to aging—to enjoy each day of his life.

Shortly after Marjory's passing, Rabbi Ed, through a series of coincidences, met up with a woman who he had known for some years and whose marriage to her husband the Rabbi had performed many years ago.

He and Jill, a speech therapist now in her late seventies, hit it off immediately. They married and he moved to the San Francisco area where she lived and they loved each other, traveled the world, wrote, dined out, and got together often with both of their families.

I cannot emphasize enough how love can bloom and our lives be enriched through having a companion who shares each moment we are given, despite the obstacles that nature puts in our way.

In May of 2015, I will be attending Ed's seventy-fifth birthday party.

My dear friend Mara Brown, a well-known writer, personal business consultant, and advisor, in her book, *The Interior Castle*, describes the fear people have of being loved and, based upon that fear and/or a previously bad relationship, "go through life living in a castle surrounded by a moat filled with alligators."

Thus, by refusing to see the potentially wonderful opportunities they may have for loving relationships, many are prevented from enjoying their life to its fullest by putting a safety net around themselves.

Happily, on the flip side, there was the story of Roz and Joe Kane (Joe passed away shortly before this book was to be published), both in their late eighties, and two of the most beautiful human beings one can have as friends. They live(d) in a facility a long distance from their adult children, who adore them. They have had numerous physical problems and have had a caregiver around the clock. They have been married for many years deeply and openly love(d) each other.

It is through their love and devotion to each other that they were able to enjoy every day of their lives together and always had smiles on their faces. They greeted all who knew them with warmth.

It is often written in song, poetry, and other communications that *one* is the loneliest number in the world. Those who are alone, particularly from mid-life on, deny themselves the opportunity to have a loving relationship and often die before they are dead.

> It's never too late to have a fling
> For autumn is just as nice as spring
> And it's never too late to fall in love.

—Me

A beautiful woman in her early seventies once told me that she and her friends had tried unsuccessfully to find senior centers and other places where women like her could find male friends and develop relationships. This is something that all communities need to address.

> "Love is the medicine for the sickness of
> mankind. We can live if we have love."

—Dr. Karl Menninger

And a bit more on the topic:

Judi and Bob are in their late eighties and have been married for sixty-four years. They have three sons and a daughter. Both of them grew up in small Texas communities. Bob's father died when Bob was very young, and he, along with Judi, struggled to educate themselves, grow in their careers, get through his time in the armed services, and raise a family.

Bob became very successful in the financial services world and was actively involved as both president and a highly recognized official in numerous major organizations.

Now, even though an aging illness confines him, he continues to offer advice and counsel to others...as he and Judi continue their love affair of over sixty years. Their goal is to keep going on with life. They are happy that their family is close to them, even though several live at a distance, and they look forward to family get-togethers.

When we see the joy that so many have sharing their last years together and read of the many tragedies that disrupt the lives of the young, it should give us the motivation to plan our journey through life early, never lose sight of the opportunities we have, and to overcome the obstacles that nature and society place in our way and enjoy every moment we are given by always being open to love.

Hm.

Hmm.

Okay. Deep breath desperately needed. One bad joke and off to the next chapter:

> Kate and Charles, a couple in their early eighties, were sitting and watching television when Kate told Charles that she was going into the kitchen to get some ice cream. Charles told her to stay where she was and that he would get it for her. He asked her what she wanted.
>
> She replied, "I want a scoop of vanilla ice cream with some chocolate syrup. On top of that I want some chopped nuts, topped with whipped cream, and chocolate chips sprinkled on that."
>
> He replied, "Okay. Vanilla ice cream with chocolate syrup topped with chopped nuts, whipped cream, and nuts."
>
> Off he went and returned ten minutes later with two scrambled eggs and bacon. She looked at what he had brought her and said, "You forgot my toast."
>
> And they lived happily ever after.
>
> These things are beautiful beyond belief:
> The pleasant weakness that comes after pain,
> The radiant greenness that comes after rain,
> The deepened faith that follow after grief,
> And the awakening to love again.
>
> —Me. Again.

SENIOR MOMENT #18

RECOGNIZING THE NEED TO GIVE UP OUR INDEPENDENCE IS CRITICAL TO LIFE'S PROCESS

One of the most difficult decisions that any person must make is that of recognition: Either they, or their companion's lifestyle and activities, may be affected by a problem with their health or physical capacity—and they need to discuss it with others involved in their life. Failure to act in a timely manner could very well make the difference between easily solving a problem or losing one's life sooner than they should.

There is after all no shame in acknowledging that you are getting older and that some of the parts could be wearing out. We all know lots of people who get a good laugh talking about these issues.

Maybe the most surprising thing that I learned in writing and researching this book was the number of family members I spoke with who live in constant fear and frustration because the person they are caring for refuses to change to accommodate a physical disability. Sadly, those same individuals are the ones who will be the ones who will end up carrying the burden when the aging person has a mishap that could have been avoided.

Sadly, those same individuals are the ones who will be the ones who will end up carrying the burden when the aging person has a mishap that could have been avoided.

We're going to get serious here, but before we do, I'll give you two bad jokes, one after the other. One is pretty funny; the other a darker groaner. You'll know which is which. And then, we'll go back to being serious.

> "A 101-year-old man and his ninety-five-year-old wife appear
> before a judge requesting a divorce after seventy-five years of
> marriage. The judge looks at them with a curious eye and asks,
> "Why did you wait so long if you've been that unhappy?

The man replies, "We wanted to wait until our children died."

—————

An elderly couple who had been married for over sixty years are in bed
when she feels him begin to run his hand up and down her body. She
became very excited because it had been some time since he had done that.

He gently moved his hand up and down her back, along her
legs, and in other delicate places, including her stomach.

He touched her buttock, the sides of her legs, and she
was really feeling good. And then he stopped.

In a soft, cuddly voice she said to him, "Darling,
that felt so good. Why did you stop?"

To which he replied, "I found the remote."

Okay? Okay. A necessary segway. Trust me.

So let's get real. As in, real serious.

Let's talk about the decision to give up your independence.

Writer John Scheibe once said, "A life is not important except in the impact it has on other lives." Truer words have never been spoken. Yes, that is my opinion.

In the aging process, either we personally recognize (although we may be in denial), or our loved ones begin to realize, that we are no longer as sharp as in previous years. Our mate in life may have passed on or be in the same situation as we are, and serious decisions must be made as to our future needs.

Certainly no person wants to give up their independence and have to rely on others. But by the same token, how fair is it to put the burden of helping get us through the journey of life on our loved ones, caregivers, and society just because we want to be free to choose our lifestyle but are no longer capable of doing so?

This issue needs to be resolved well in advance of the event which, should it arise, can indeed have a reasonably satisfying conclusion if planned for prudently. By the time we reach our fifties, we need to have begun to openly discuss, with our family caregivers and medical professionals, all of the issues that could affect our lives as the aging process takes its natural course. (Actually, given the number of deaths that occur early in life, we need to do this well before the age of fifty.)

As an example, very recent statistics suggest that Alzheimer's is one of the diseases that apparently begins to raise its head as early as when we reach our fifties.

My own years of experience as a trained caregiver, as well as knowledge gained from speaking with others, clearly identifies acceptance as one of the most important and yet least considered issues facing us in our lifetime.

> "When a father gives to his son, they both laugh.
> When a son gives to his father, they both cry."

—Rabbi Joseph Telushkin
Yiddish Proverb
Jewish Wisdom

The Most Difficult Decision

Whatever your personal situation—married, single, living alone, with another person or with your parents—a decision has to be made as to how the rest of your life will be lived, and with whom. As traumatic as this is for each individual, just stop and consider the effect it has on those who care for us, even if they do not live with us or are at a great distance away.

Most of all, if you don't plan (that word again) now and have several contingency plans in those prepared to be involved in your care pass away, you will be in serious trouble later on.

Tsuris, as we say in Yiddish.

In the 1930s, during the Great Depression, families in the United States lived close to each other and helped take care of the elderly and sick amongst them. In fact, in my case, because Grandma was living with us and literally aging and dying in the next room, we experienced the life and death process each day.

A bit of history: Things were different "back then." Period.

With the growth of governmental programs (such as Medicare), the expansion of care centers, and the mobility of our population, significant changes have occurred which at once removed the daily in-home experience and transferred it to remote locations. This has now placed a great burden on our economy, society, and families.

The vast distances that many of us live from our aging loved ones puts a major mental, financial, and moral strain on all of us. More and more families are faced with having to decide if they need to move closer to where their aging loved one lives, or if the aging person needs to be uprooted and moved to where the family is—placing them into a community where they have no roots.

Another major issue involved in giving up our independence is that of driving. Each day, we hear of elderly persons being involved in fatal accidents. And, more often than not, it is a passenger(s) in the car being driven by that person who is killed, or seriously injured.

What is most sad about this is that the family, the aging driver's doctors, and all of those who know them are afraid to broach the subject, or do anything about it usually until it is too late.

I personally witnessed an accident that took the lives of three persons, one of whom (the driver), unbeknownst to me at the time, was the eighty-one-year-old mother of a friend. She lost control of the vehicle. If you want to kill yourself fine, but don't kill me.

More reality…

There is a very sweet and loving person living in the Independent Living Center in Southern California who has such dementia that he often cannot find the way around the facility and does not know what day it is. Nevertheless, that person is legally responsible for the financial affairs of a friend, who lives in a similar facility.

What then?

When I investigated the reasoning behind this, I was told that the friends and family of the person being helped wanted nothing to do with those matters, and that the family of the individual who was legally responsible did not want to aggravate the helper by removing that responsibility—even though they could be liable for any negatives that came out of what was being done.

"A wise person plans ahead to ensure they will be traveling on a smooth highway."

—Me

SENIOR MOMENT #19

AS WE DEAL WITH OUR AGING OR SERIOUS ILLNESS ISSUES, OUR FAMILIES NEED US AS MUCH AS WE NEED THEM

No one can deny that discussing life and death issues can be most difficult. Individuals and their loved ones would do anything to not have to open up the subject, but the fact is that at the end of life, everyone will find it much easier to deal with all of the issues involved if a plan is agreed upon and in place.

So how and when do you begin?

While working with the Northridge Medical Center Hospice in 1994, I was asked to visit with Alex, a Brooklyn-born and raised man in his seventies who was being challenged by terminal Cancer.

He and his wife, a very caring woman who worked as a textbook representative, lived in an apartment complex which, coincidentally, was the scene of massive destruction and death during the 1994 earthquake.

His wife had told me that they had two sons who lived not too far away and that they were having a great struggle with Alex because he refused to speak with them about his illness, his feelings about life, and all of the other issues that have been discussed throughout this book.

After spending several hours with him, during which time I carefully explained why I was there and asking him some basic questions, I quickly realized that my task was not going to be easy. His wife was beside herself and was near a breakdown because she and the family were being totally rejected by Alex.

I left contemplating my next move. The next day I received a call from his wife who told me that Alex did not wish to see me again. If you've paid attention so far, you know that I am not one who gives up easily.

The following day I called and asked to speak to him. I said, "I want to take you to lunch tomorrow and talk with you further. If after that you do not want ever to see me again, I will go away." He reluctantly agreed, and I arranged to pick him up and take him to a restaurant close to where he lived.

As we were seated he said to me, "What do you want? I grew up on the streets of Brooklyn, and I know people like you. You are trying to take my wife. You cannot have her. You are after my money and my car. You cannot have them. Everybody is after something in life, and you are no different."

I told him that I wanted none of those things and that my purpose in life was to help others like him when they have a need. I explained that his family was totally frustrated with him and his refusal to speak to them about his feelings, his illness, and how he felt about life and death. We spoke about the fact that his sons no longer wanted to visit him and why, and we discussed that his wife feared coming home from work at night. Finally, I suggested that if he could not find it within himself to speak directly with the family, that he should ask them to get a tape recorder and open himself up through that device.

The next day his wife called me crying on the phone. She asked me what happened when we had lunch. I asked her why and she said that when she got home last night Alex was sitting on the bed crying. He asked her to buy him a tape recorder and then the two of them sat up all night crying and speaking about his situation.

As we reach our fifties we need start sharing our thoughts about life and death with our loved ones. One way to do this is to begin to share your feelings on what aspects of life give you the most meaning. Also, discuss how your religious or spiritual beliefs—if any—affect your feelings about dying and death in general.

By sharing these end-of-life issues with your loved ones, you will not only increase chances of your wishes being followed, but also of responses to other questions too, such as: How important is it to you to be physically independent and stay in your home? What are the down sides of that? Particularly, how it would affect those who are responsible for your care. Finally, if the situation were presented, would you prefer to die at home?

Such an honest discussion will help immensely in reducing the mental anxiety of all of those who love and support you. And, at the same time, as painful as it is those loved ones need to stop, take deep breaths, and recognize the depth of the pain, they too must accept that their lives will change as well.

Without meaning to be redundant, it is most important that all parties involved in this discussion need to not only be in total agreement, but also need to understand that it is the caregivers who will be carrying the burden—and their needs outweigh yours. Truly.

Remember that. Without the caregivers, you just may be in deep doo-doo.

During this discussion, which importantly needs to be reviewed from time to time as conditions change, it is wise to speak about what prompted your thoughts, such as an article you had read, watching others go though serious illnesses, and death, etc.

In addition, the following steps need to be taken to make the journey as smooth as possible. Be sure to also seek the advice and help of qualified professionals if you feel you need to.

For now:

1. **Get estate planning immediately underway.** Plan legally for your possible incapacity by preparing documents such as a durable power of attorney, a healthcare power of attorney, and a living will along with a will or trust. Be certain that your loved ones have copies of all documents and know where the originals are stored.

2. **Consolidate and organize medical history and related information.** Among the most important steps that can be taken is to be certain that you have a well-documented, organized record of all of your healthcare records, including medicines, tests, and surgeries. Also, keep notes on medicines that did not work for you and what reactions you had. Keep these in an easily accessible binder, an online tools such as "Life Ledger" or USB drives.

3. **Keep records of personal family medical history.** Oftentimes, this information is invaluable when we incur medical problems and our doctors can have the information they need in order to treat us more effectively.

There is a woman in her early eighties who lives alone in a small community many miles from her family. She lost her husband awhile back and has no close relatives and a small handful of friends. Her health, including her physical abilities, are failing, but she refuses to accept that and will not consider moving to a new city near her family. She insists that her family is too busy to take care of her, and besides, it would take her over a year to get ready to make a move.

When she is told that it would be much more difficult on her family to have to travel to help her, she rejects that argument, as she does when told that it's time that she think only about the burden she is placing on her loved ones by not making the move.

As difficult as it is for one to make this kind of decision, when the time comes it really is the only choice one has, and the earlier it is made the better everyone will be.

SENIOR MOMENT #20

UNDERSTANDING WHAT CARE FACILITIES ARE AVAILABLE

Let's do something different. Let's *begin* with a bad joke as opposed to ending with one. They say, "Variety is the spice of life." Right?

So...

> Three elderly single women living in a retirement home are sitting by the pool one sunny afternoon, when a gentleman in his late seventies appears and jumps in. One of the women looks at him and asks, in a loud voice, "Are you new here? We haven't seen you before…"
>
> He responds in the affirmative. One of the other women then asks: "Where did you come from?"
>
> He responds by saying, "I was in prison for twenty-five years for killing my wife."
>
> The third women exclaims with great joy: "So, you are single!"

Okay, I'm better than that. I know, I know…

As the aging process moves forward and we or our loved one requires part-time or full-time assistance, there are many choices to choose from, each with their unique pluses and minuses. It is important that we take the time to carefully look at which one best suits the needs of all concerned.

Such as:

Homecare Agencies vs. Independent Care Providers

In situations where the person with needs can safely live at home, there are numerous agencies which provide full- or part-time qualified and trained caregivers. You must first be certain that the agency you select has a good reputation and is qualified to not only provide qualified caregivers, but also to advise you on all matters relating to your present (and future) needs.

Regardless of the age of the person requiring a home health caregiver, it is important from both a comfort level and legal point of view that those making the decision carefully consider the many issues involved and ask the right questions.

Hopefully, plans are not made in the midst of an emergency situation and there is enough time to make the proper preparations for the patient's care. Yes, there will be times when emergency situations occur, but nevertheless, during the process these matters must be clarified and adjustments made.

For example, my beloved Anna's doctor called me at nine p.m. on a Thursday night to inform me that she was going to be sent home from the hospital the very next day. Based upon information previously provided, it was my understanding that she was going to be sent to a care facility. Well, that changed very quickly.

We had exactly twelve hours to empty our bedroom, set it up as a hospital room, and hire a caregiver. I was able to do so because I had spent weeks investigating what actions needed to be taken in such a situation.

Please note that not all states require home health agencies to be licensed and, in fact, many states do not provide for licensing at all. California is one of those states.

It is important, then, when choosing a qualified home health care agency that the agency, at a minimum, possesses a current business license, proof of Worker's Compensation insurance, and liability insurance, including theft coverage (known as "Bonding"). Also, they must provide you with specifics on their nurses' aides and W-2 employees of the agency.

Questions To Ask:

1. Is the individual and/or agency licensed, insured, and bonded? Once you or your family hire them, if they do not meet all of the immigration regulations (many healthcare professionals are not U.S. Citizens but have "right to work" authorization and Social

Security verification, and can be legally hired but do not meet tax requirements) you could be held responsible for paying their taxes.

Note, too, that there are professional care providers from countries outside the U.S. who have been trained as nurses, medical assistants and doctors who can only work as non-medical or custodial caregivers until they receive proper U.S. licensing.

2. Has the caregiver told you that they are an independent contractor and requested payment in cash? If so, you are then liable for any safety and medical issues or injuries that may be incurred by them, as well as disability lawsuits or assault claims.

3. Have you seen their tax returns to ensure that they are filing their 1099 Tax Forms? In California, as well as many other states, you could be liable for the applicable taxes if they in fact are not paying them. Keep in mind that there may be no statute of limitations and this could be very costly to you.

4. Does the Agency treat their caregivers as employees or independent contractors? If they do not consider them employees then you may be held responsible for their taxes and Workers Compensation payment.

Your Caregivers and You

When choosing an agency as a healthcare provider, it is important to select one whose hiring practices include a requirement that their caregivers have a minimum of three years of current caregiving experience, and that they are skilled to perform any or all of the following tasks:

a) Assistance with bathing, dressing, toileting (including incontinence care);

b) Monitoring blood pressure;

c) Oxygen intake monitoring;

d) Transferring and assistance from bed to wheelchair or commode. Use of Hoyer lift when necessary;

e) Bedridden Care and Repositioning Techniques;

f) Range of Motion Exercise;

g) Gait Supervision and Shadowing; bed to wheelchair or commode. ;

h) Alzheimer's & Dementia Communication and Redirection;

i) Nutrition and Hydration expertise for Diabetics, Heart Patients, and other conditions which require restrictive diets.

They may also provide some or all of the following optional services:

1. Meal Planning and Preparation

2. Transportation to doctors and other elated needs-as well as proper insurance for these services.

3. Light Housekeeping.

4. Medication Reminders

5. Hospital Sitting.

6. Live-Out and Live-In Care.

Two other issues of importance are language compatibility. Is the assigned caregiver able to clearly communicate with the person being cared for? Also, is the patient comfortable with the age and personality of the caregiver? If not, you must understand how the agency will resolve that matter. On several occasions, in the middle of the night, I had to fire a caregiver from a hospice who was giving our very competent caregiver a difficult time. Personality differences and mood changes can seriously affect the relationship between the patient and the caregiver.

By all means, be certain that you meet and are comfortable with the management of the agency and have a clear understanding of their communication processes. You must ensure that they are available to you at all times, including when problems arise and other unanticipated issues get in the way of taking care of your loved one. The caregiver also needs to clearly understand that no matter what the patient's moods, they are not to be harsh with them.

When or if it is no longer feasible to keep the patient at home with a home companion, and a home away from home is required, it is important to carefully, with the advice of all of those involved, determine what kind of facilities are available and how they can best serve your needs.

Obviously this also involves a financial commitment. It is therefore necessary to look into all of the additional costs—both real and hidden—in making the decision as to how best to proceed.

In choosing a facility, always keep the following in mind:

1. Do not make your selection based upon the food being served. Under the best conditions, food served in "institutional-type facilities" is not going to be like you cooked at home or that which is served in restaurants.

2. It is institutional and needs to meet the needs of a wide variety of health situations, such as salt-free diets, diabetic and gastrointestinal needs, etc.

3. Be sure you understand the transportation services such as shopping, medical appointments, etc., provided by the facility and if they charge extra for them.

4. Look into the type of activities provided to the residents to be certain they are compatible with your needs. Not only should the activities be inside the facility, but outside events are important as well.

5. If it is a medically approved unit, you need to determine if your doctor goes to that facility.

6. Clearly understand whether the facility is licensed, and for what.

7. Ask about the training and licensing of the staff.

8. Your changing physical condition may necessitate moving from one facility to another.

9. Spend time meeting the residents of the facility and evaluating their physical and mental capabilities. While the residents may have been wonderfully warm and compassionate persons during their pre-aging days, be aware of the fact that aging often changes one's personality.

10. Finally, be cognizant of the fact that no matter what type of facility one moves into, it takes a while to fit into the population and understand the personalities and social interaction that occurs among those who are aging.

Breathe.

We have just passed some information-heavy section.

A heavy section, period.

So breathe.

Breathe, as we enter another.

And we'll get back to joking later. I promise.

The end stages of life, you see, are not *always* a laughing matter.

And we go on. Did you really think we were done?

Not yet. As for the rest…

One of the most important decisions we need to make early in life is how are we going to pay for the care we need as we grow older. Investing early in life and purchasing the right kind of life insurance to protect our families, saving accounts and many other methods are certainly important, but as I myself found out (without realizing it at the time of purchase), long-term healthcare policies are critical in addressing this issue.

Because people are living longer, these policies are becoming harder to get and more costly as well; however, I cannot emphasize enough the benefits that can accrue by making them a priority choice.

Adult Daytime Health Care

This is an adult day service that offers comprehensive health and social support services. Typically, such facilities will provide on-site nurses, therapists, social workers and other health professionals. They also may provide programs that include a mixture of health and social support services for older adults, for periods of twenty-four hours or less.

Alzheimer's Facilities

These are licensed facilities or special care units within a larger facility which may also contain other care units for less-confined individuals. These facilities usually provide intermediate nursing, medical, and rehabilitation care in a safe and controlled environment for individuals who have been diagnosed with Alzheimer's disease or dementia.

Assisted Living Facilities

These facilities maximize an individual's ability to live independently and receive a lower level of assistance than skilled nursing and other facilities that provide major assistance programs. They (usually) provide twenty-four hour on-call assistance and personal and home care assistance, including bathing, dressing, meals, and housekeeping.

Note: Some of the aforementioned facilities do include special dementia care units under their umbrella and will provide assistance with feeding, range-of-motion supervision, and a higher level of personal care assistance. Be aware, however, that Medicare does not generally cover care in these units, and the population can include persons with beginning stages of memory loss and other physical and mental impairments. Also, recent changes in governmental healthcare programs—which kicked off in 2015—are going to have a significant effect on the cost of home medical care workers. This will make it even more difficult for many to get the kind of care they need but cannot afford.

Note, too, that it is also important in looking into this kind of facility to determine if they are licensed for medical care. Most are not, and this could be a problem in case of emergency needs.

Onward.

Board and Care Homes

These are residential-oriented facilities usually offering a light level of care for up to ten individuals in a home-like atmosphere. They may not be licensed or certified and may also be referred to as Residential Care Facilities.

Convalescent Home AKA Skilled Nursing Facilities (SNF)

State-licensed facilities that provide a safe, therapeutic environment for individuals who require rehabilitative care or no longer can live independently due to a functional or cognitive impairment.

Once again, always take the time to visit these facilities and ascertain whether you are comfortable with the atmosphere, staff attitude, and the services they provide. Often, there are a number of patients sharing rooms, and many persons have mental impairments which cause them to keep their roommates from getting proper sleep.

Residential Care Homes

Such facilities offer personal care and individual attention to older adults, persons with disabilities, and others whose limitations prevent them from living alone.

These facilities generally provide a room, meals, and supervision. They may also specialize in specific needs such as Alzheimer's or developmental disabilities. Again, you want to be sure you are looking into a licensed facility.

Respite Care

Such homes provide temporary or intermittent care for individuals with functional or cognitive impairments that provide relief to caregivers from the demands of ongoing care. This care can be provided in the home, in the community, or overnight at the facility.

Retirement Communities

Often referred to as "Senior 55+ Housing or 55+ Apartment Communities, they provide shelter and support services to older adults who are nearly or totally independent. Their services may include housekeeping, meal preparation, and social, as well as recreational activities and transportation.

Skilled Nursing Facility (SNF)

Sometimes referred to as Nursing Homes, or Convalescent Homes. These are state-licensed facilities which provide a safe, therapeutic environment for individuals who require rehabilitative care and can no longer live independently.

Hospice Care

When a doctor determines that a person is in the end-stage of life, hospice care usually is recommended. Such services provided are tailored to the specific needs of the individual. Whether the patient is at home or in some of the above-mentioned facilities, your medical team will advise you as to what is required.

Phew! Not all that much fun pondering your old age now, is it?

SENIOR MOMENT #21

EVERY AGING PERSON NEEDS AN ADVOCATE

"Growing old is like being increasingly penalized
for a crime you have not committed."

—Anthony Powell

The need for an advocate.

When we are going though any kind of a physical or mental problem, either in our own home or in a facility and are under a doctor's care or even hospice, it is important that someone close to us—either family or friend—is fully informed as to our care and treatment. Why? Because more often than not there are disagreements as to what is supposed to be done and by whom. For example:

1. The administration of medications may be confusing due to the need to often make changes. Your "advocate"—a helper of some sort—needs to clearly understand the doctor's up-to-date instructions and resolve any conflict, because more often than not the caregiver may not be clear or may not have been updated.

2. During Anna's last few weeks, she developed an infection and was running a fever. The doctor's instructions to me were that if her temperature rose to 101 degrees, she was to be given a specific medicine, but the caregiver had misunderstood the instructions and refused to give it. As her advocate, I had to call the doctor and confirm what I understood to be the facts.

3. Diet issues can also cause disagreements among caregivers. Sometimes the patient wants certain foods and their caregiver will not give those to them, only to have the patient react badly. In looking at the reasons, it is frequently discovered that the instructions the caregiver looked at was not current.

4. Issues regarding sleep hours, personal care, ambulatory needs and related matters can affect decisions being made on the patient's behalf.

5. Anna had an accumulation of fluid in her lungs that required draining every three days. On occasion, a visiting nurse checked her after two days and said there was no fluid and we needed to wait four days. That was erroneous, and she began to have serious breathing problems. I had to call the doctor who immediately sent another nurse out to clear the lungs.

The reason for an advocate is to ensure that the person in charge of your care has communicated properly with those who are administrating that care. Having a person very close to you during an illness is absolutely critical to proper and efficient care. Never assume that the caregiver—even hospital staff members—always have the correct information. Be safe, not sorry.

—⊰•⊱—

As I learned myself, not once but three times, just after you reach fifty years of age there is a major reason why it is essential that you select a person close to you to be your advocate in case of illness, accidents, or just the aging process.

Hospitals and care centers are very busy and often the staff is working under highly pressurized conditions. Individuals have a very difficult time getting personalized attention, and this adds to their already stressful situation.

Another major issue of concern in this regard is that when a person, particularly an aging one, is placed in any kind of a care or medical facility, they are more often than not treated not as an adult, but as a dependent child. And even though the staff are dedicated and understand their role, they often erect a wall between their professional work and the personal concerns and fears of the patient. This creates a terrible situation for the patient and leaves them angry, frustrated, and alone.

By having a loved one close by—someone who can get them the attention they so urgently need—is invaluable and can make all the difference in their comfort level.

During Anna's final journey, my doctors advised me that I had the need to have surgery on an artery in my right leg. I was told that it would be a relatively simple procedure done in the surgeon's office and that the recovery would only be a few days.

Things didn't quite pan our as planned. A friend took me to the clinic and then home after the procedure, Unfortunately, the nerve in my leg was damaged, and two days after the procedure I was rushed to the hospital in severe pain.

Since Anna obviously was not there to help and my children all live many miles from my home, I was in the hospital by myself, in terrific pain and thinking only about my wife. My doctors were not always available and the staff of the facility was less than helpful.

I had no one there to advocate for me.

As it has turned out, after over a year of seeing the best specialists in the country and going through all kinds of tests—as well as trying every known pain medication—the problem is not solvable and the severe pain remains. Walking has become increasingly difficult.

I finally came to the conclusion that I either had to ignore the pain and live my life as normally as possible, or become a total invalid sitting in a wheelchair. I chose life and decided to live with the pain. That has proven to be a very wise decision.

I frequently compare the above case to my earlier experience in 1989, when I was advised at the age of sixty that unless I had surgery for my Crohn's disease, for which I was diagnosed in 1964 that I would shortly die.

Anna was with me throughout that long and difficult surgery and recovery and acted superbly as my advocate. She made it so easy for me to go through the process.

As a result of this experience, I later became President of the San Fernando Chapter of the Crohn's Colitis Foundation of America (CCFA). I was working with a wonderful group of persons who either had, or were involved with, others who were challenged by this debilitating disease. In my role I did public seminars and raised money to support research for a cure. Kelsey Grammer, the actor and comedian, assisted me with that project.

Finally, for this section, please indulge me as I add one more case study.

Sharon was an unmarried retired schoolteacher, in her early seventies, living in Southern California. She had two younger sisters who lived in different cities some distance from her.

She was in the early stages of pancreatic cancer.

I had just moved back to California and lived near her. I was a volunteer hospice caregiver working with the Orange County, California Nursing Association, and was asked by the office to visit Sharon and see what help we could provide her.

The Association volunteers all wore badges with their names on them. Mine said "Bernie." When I visited Sharon for the first time, one of her sisters was also visiting. I spent an hour with Sharon and then arranged to follow up on a weekly basis.

The next day, the office called me and told me that Sharon's sister had called and, at Sharon's request, I was not to see her again. Naturally I was baffled, but I did not make an issue out of it.

Two weeks later the office called again. They told me that both sisters were visiting Sharon and they wanted me to call and help them with a problem that Sharon had. I made an appointment and went to the home, where I was met outside by both women who apologized for asking me not to come back. They explained that they had a sister named Bernice who had died recently, and that when Sharon saw my name tag "Bernie," it reminded her of her late sister. They asked me to remove my nametag, which I did. They then asked me to help take Sharon to her doctor, as he would not make a house call. I did so as well and continued to spend time with her.

Sharon's sisters were her advocates, and advocates play a key role in the care of their loved ones.

Even in issues as seemingly minor (but are not) as name badges.

> "The great secret that all old people share is that you haven't
> changed in seventy to eighty, only your body has."
>
> —Anonymous

Larry, a friend, was a public employee in his fifties being challenged by lung cancer. His wife was a prominent businessperson who was in total denial about her husband's illness. They had no children.

Larry's wife wanted nothing to do with his treatment, nor decisions relating to it. She left early each day to go to work and returned each night after dinner. He was under the care of hospice and his neighbors were helping as best they could.

Coincidentally, I was asked by hospice to deliver luncheon speeches about our programs; one of those speeches was to a women's business group.

When I arrived at the event I noticed a woman walking out of the room. I recognized her as being his wife from a photo I had seen in his home.

My talk was about the advocacy issue and other hospice care matters. About halfway through my talk, I noticed Larry's wife coming back into to room and standing near the doorway.

When I had finished speaking and was about to sit down, she came over to me and said, "I don't know if you know who I am. I am Larry's wife."

I acknowledged that I did know that, and she walked away.

Later that afternoon, when I was back in my office, I received a phone call from the hospice office and was asked by the executive who called me, "What did you do today?" When I told her about speaking to the group she said, "No, you were building bridges."

When I asked her to explain, she told me that Larry's wife had called the office crying and apologized for being so insensitive to his needs. She asked the office to tell her what she needed to do to take care of him.

Larry lived for another year and a half, with his wife at his side, making certain that he had the care required in the time he had left.

> "Love is not something we give to others only in good
> times, but most importantly in difficult times as well."

—Me

I Got a Million of 'Em.

Jokes. Bad jokes, that is.

I don't want you to be weighed down by the heaviness of all this as you progress through this book. Aging ain't pretty, and neither is my humor.

Nor my age spots, nor my wrinkles…

To that end, let's take another brief break and share some pretty awful gags (that hopefully will make you laugh uproariously as we prepare for the end):

—◆◆◆—

A police officer pulls over an elderly woman for speeding while she drives her husband to an appointment. The officer tries to explain the reason he pulled her over, but she keeps turning to her husband asking, "Huh? What did he just say?"

The husband says, "He said he stopped you for speeding."

The officer asks her for her driver's license. Again, she turns to her husband and asks, "What did he say?"

The husband replies, "He wants to see your driver's license."

She hands it to him and he notices that she is from Brownsville.

He says that he remembers that city well, and, in fact, he had the worst sexual experience of his life there.

The woman again turns to her husband and asks, "What did he say?"

The husband replies to her, "He said he thinks he knows you."

—◆◆◆—

An eighty-year-old man is lying in bed, near-death. His wife of fifty years is at his bedside. He opens his eyes and says to her, "You know, Ida, I was just thinking. When I got pneumonia several years ago, you were at my side taking care of me. And when I had my open-heart surgery last year, you were at my side taking care of me. Now that I have prostate cancer, once again, you are at my side taking care of me. Ida…I think you are bad luck!"

Rimspot! Okay, just one more before you throw me out of the room:

Phil, an insurance salesman in his late-seventies, stops at a shopping center on his way home from work. He has decided to purchase some flowers for his wife of many years, Nancy, who is in her mid-seventies. As he leaves the flower shop he notices a candy store. He goes in and purchases her a box of truffles as well.

When he gets home, his hands full of goodies, he rings the bell. Nancy opens the door. When she sees what Phil is carrying she begins to cry, whereupon Phil asks, "Why the tears?"

She says, "This has been a terrible day. I dropped my favorite cake plate and it broke. I was supposed to have lunch with some friends, but they got sick and cancelled. Our telephone system was messed up and it took me almost all day to get in touch with the phone repair service, AND NOW YOU COME HOME DRUNK!!!"

Thank you, ladies and gents. I play Vegas next week.

SENIOR MOMENT #22

MEDICAL ALERT SYSTEMS ARE ESSENTIAL TO THE SAFETY OF THE ELDERLY

Why have I written this book?

Just because.

No kidding.

Because despite the crust, despite the oft-bizarre jabs at old-age humor (which I sincerely hope you don't find *that* bad)… I care.

I care that you plan. And I care that you really are well prepared and ready for when the day comes. If not the day for you, then for your loved ones.

This is me, unfettered. Bernard Seymour Otis.

Just because…I really do care.

That is all.

On Medical Alerts and Companionship

At the time of my seventieth birthday, Anna and I decided it would be wise to install a medical alert system in our home just in case an emergency arose. She was sixty years of age and we were both vibrant and active individuals. Little did we realize at that time how important our decision would be during her illness.

A year later, during Anna's second year of cancer treatment when we were preparing to go to a doctor's appointment and leave our housekeeper to finish her task, our telephone rang and shattered any semblance of security. Emergency service informed me that they had received a signal that someone had fallen in our home.

Louisa (our housekeeper) and I quickly ran to the master bathroom and found Anna lying on the floor. Paramedics were quickly dispatched; Anna was taken to the hospital and then spent two months in rehab. Had we not had the system in place there is no telling what might have resulted—but I had her for another year.

There are many such systems available, but whichever one you choose, be certain it has a immediate call to your home and an immediate paramedic alert, and by all means give the system the names and phone numbers for alternative contacts. Also, make sure those contacts have easy access to your home.

Do not assume just because more than one person lives in that home that if an accident happens that the others will be there or know that such an event took place.

It is wise to carefully look into all of the issues raised in this and other chapters of the book before making a decision as to how and where we or our loved ones are cared for, but always discuss this with your primary doctors and be certain that you know if and how your physician will available to continue treatment in the chosen facility.

> "Aging is a life-spanning process of growth and development
> from birth to death. Old age is an integral part of the whole,
> bringing fulfillment and self-actualization. I regard aging
> as a triumph, a result of strength and survivorship"

—Margaret Kuhn

A Note from the Author

When the title of this book was selected, including the words, "If You Were Not Born Into a Wealthy Family," the intent was to inject some humor into it. Unfortunately, there is also a great deal of truth to the use of those words as well.

As the population of aging individuals rapidly grows, the number of care facilities per capita shrinks, the need for more well-trained and managed home caregivers rises. The cost of maintaining them also soars, and we are faced with a major financial crisis in the healthcare industry.

In addition to the issue of immigration as it affects healthcare workers, —a large majority of them are immigrants with legal status—home health agencies and care facilities are faced with tight budgets, and, as a result of 2015 changes in federal minimum pay regulations, will have even higher costs. Due to this, the question becomes how will they—and for that matter, *we*—be able to meet the financial burden?

During my research I interviewed dozens of caregivers in various facilities, as well as home caregivers, and their stories are all pretty much the same.

Lara is a forty-five-year-old Russian immigrant who has been legally in this country for three years. She is married and has a grown son. Her husband works as a day laborer.

Lara is employed as a trained caregiver in a very well-known caregiving facility. She is employed on a part-time basis at a minimum wage so that the facility will not have to pay overtime and benefits. This requires her to work several jobs and very long hours just to maintain a low-level life style.

Her employers all have the same financial problem and in order to stay solvent and be able to attract residents, they need to have a tight control of their budgets.

Is there a better reason why it is so important to plan early and be prepared?

Even if you are not from this country.

While attending the University of Michigan, I had three friends from high school who attended and were also majoring in engineering. One night while having dinner at a favorite watering hole, the Pretzel Bell, they were discussing the human body and how it came to be formed.

One of them said that if you look at it closely and observe the way the joints are put together, it is obvious that it was designed by a mechanical engineer.

Howard then said that he believed that, because of the way the nervous system was put together, it had to have been done by an electrical engineer.

Don completely disagreed and speculated that only a civil engineer would run a toxic pipeline through a recreational area.

The point is, we don't know. Neither do our trained caregivers. But, likely, they know more than you. Respect them and work with them, even if they do not share your language.

SENIOR MOMENT #23

FINDING WAYS TO DEAL WITH THE LOSS OF SIGHT

"One should never count the years. One should instead count one's interests. I have kept young trying never to lose my childhood sense of wonderment. I am glad I still have a vivid curiosity about the world I live in."

—Helen Keller

I've said it before: Sight may be the most important sense of all as it, more often than not, has the most effect on our daily lives and activities.

Losing the ability to see what is going on around us—to look at those we love, to watch as our children, grandchildren and great grandchildren grow—is devastating.

In addition, when we are ill and have hours and hours of time alone, the inability to read, watch television, or just sit in the outdoors and look at the moon, sun, and stars is difficult to endure.

Because my beloved Anna was well known for her work with the blind, I had the opportunity to speak with, learn from, and be involved with blind persons of all ages. In fact, during her last five years of life, following her retirement from the State Department of Rehabilitation for the Blind, Anna conducted special seminars for aging blind persons for the Center for the Visually Impaired in Los Angeles.

There are many stories I could tell about professionals actively involved in their daily activities who suddenly, in their middle-to-late ages, begin to lose their eyesight, but first let me share my personal experiences with the subject of vision impairment and blindness.

Many years ago while working my way through college, I was employed by a large credit department store, Peoples Outfitting Company, in downtown Detroit. One of the owners, the Wineman family's son-in-law Henry Moses, had a son who was blind.

Henry used to drive me to work, and on one of our trips he told me about the home he had just built that had no corners in it; all rooms were rounded so that there was no obstacle for his son as he moved about the house.

Further, Henry and his family were all trained to deal with the blindness issue by going into the basement of the home, where there was no light, and blindfolding themselves for hours on end so that they could better understand the world of their son.

Ironically, when she lived in England during her twenty-year marriage, Anna worked for the Jewish Blind Society of London, where she became well known as specialist with the blind and she told me that she had learned this same technique and practiced it in her work.

Steve Wynn, the well-known Las Vegas Hotel/Casino entrepreneur, has had macular disintegration for well over sixty years. He founded a large foundation doing research on that disease, and yet he has successfully built an empire in the gaming industry and made a major contribution to helping those with vision problems find ways to live their lives happily and productively.

From the time that Steve and his family moved to Las Vegas in the mid 1960s, they worked tirelessly to ensure that those with vision problems had the resources they needed to travel life's road. We should all be most grateful to them for their contribution to life.

There are many ways in which individuals with vision problems can get the help and support they need in order to compensate for the difficulties they have. All over the country there are organizations like the Braille Institute, Center for the Visually Impaired, and others that conduct seminars, in-home training programs and other types of programs to help those of any age, with sight problems.

Also, many of these organizations create large-print books, books on tape, and other vehicles of aid to further make life comfortable for the blind.

After her retirement from her position with State of California, Anna held weekly seminars for the Center for the Partially Sighted (as well as blind) on all kinds of worldly issues which the attendees had interest in.

Quite often I was asked to speak to these groups about my writings and work in the food and beverage industry. I always felt good about doing so because of the enthusiastic reception I received.

Many of those who attended these sessions had been blind since birth or were gradually losing their eyesight, but nevertheless were active in life, or finding ways to be so through the help of all of those in this specialized field who were working hard and under often difficult conditions to help them do so.

Wherever you live, there is a group out there ready to help make your life that much better by showing you ways to live with your sight problems.

To a person who has been born with any kind of physical impairment, living life is a normal thing. While they certainly need all of the love, help, and encouragement to get through each day, to one who suddenly loses the ability to see or function physically, it is a frightening experience.

SENIOR MOMENT #24

KNOWING YOUR MEANING OF LIFE CONTRIBUTES TO A HAPPY JOURNEY

We've spent nearly a lifetime together in this book! Really. I'm not trying to be funny… for a change.

So, if we're truly in the "nitty-gritty," as I say…

What has been the meaning of your life?

If you cannot yet answer, you may want to ask yourself the following question:

If you knew that this was going to be your last day of life, how would you spend it?

Your answer will help you with clarity.

As for me:

If I knew when I was going to die, I would get up on my last day, and I would:

- Tell my close family and friends how much I love them,
- Help a person(s) in need,
- Do something that I always enjoyed, and
- Return to my home and spend my last hours in the arms of the woman with whom I have an emotional and meaningful love.

But even if I did not know this was going to be my last day, this is how I want to live so as to have a happy and meaningful life until the end.

See what I mean? It's all about clarity.

If four years ago someone had asked me what my meaning in life was, no doubt I would have replied that it was to continue my career, take care of my health, share my love with Anna, live a good life, help others, and watch, with joy, as my children and grandchildren matured and went on to success.

Soon after her passing, I moved into an assisted living center where I quickly reinforced my belief about the meaning of life, as I lived in a community of wonderful human beings—many of whom had memory problems, physical disabilities, and other difficulties, which left them with meaningless lives and lost in a world where they are just waiting for the end.

Every word that appears at the top of this chapter comes from my heart, and I believe that each person as they reach this period of life can feel life's meaningfulness, just as a blind person who cannot see can feel love and does so on a daily basis.

Instead, her last years turned into a nightmare for me and I suddenly realized that there was much more to life than those simplistic desires, as important as they are. It was at the very moment that I was told about Anna's ultimate fate, that I stopped and asked myself, "What is my purpose in life?"

The answer was obvious, and for the most part, it is exactly what I had been self- consciously doing since my father planted the seed in my mind many years earlier. It is also what Viktor E. Frankl himself wrote: "The purpose in life is to help others find theirs."

I needed to help my beloved deal with her pain and challenges. I needed to overcome my own weaknesses so that I could better serve others. I needed to prepare myself for the end of the journey so as not to be a burden on others. Above all else, I needed to help others heal the wounds incurred during life's journey so that they could find the meaning of their own lives.

In the previous pages of this book you have been given a great deal of information about the journey through life and the many issues you need to consider as you make the trip.

It is sad to watch so many of those we love and care for suddenly finding themselves, along with their families, faced with the realization that death is inevitable. It is sad to see them finding themselves so unprepared.

Death is, without question, a sad subject which nobody wants to discuss, but one which we all will sooner or later need to be prepared for. Therefore, doesn't it make sense to talk about it and make plans to deal with it before it is suddenly thrust upon us and creates chaos for everyone involved?

And also, doesn't it make sense to discuss how we can go on enjoying life to its fullest and not die before our time by planning ahead and setting realistic goals for doing just that when the aging process begins to take its toll?

Each day we should be able to get up, open the blinds, look up at the sky, and enjoy the freshness of the air and be thankful for all that we have been given.

Recently, a friend asked me if I was ready to die. Up until that moment, the truth is that I really had not given a great deal of thought to it. Over the next few days I seriously pondered the question, and my answer is "yes."

I know my time will come and that other than taking reasonable care of myself and moderating my activities, there is not much control I have over it—so why worry about it (as I like to counsel others)?

No two people should worry about the same thing.

So, while I take each moment of life as it comes, I will leave the details of my life's end for God to worry about.

Probably the most profound words that I know on this subject were written by one of, if not the, most respected Judaic scholars and teachers, Rabbi Joshua Heschel, in his volume *Man is Not Alone*.

"The deepest wisdom man can attain is to know that his destiny is to aid, to serve. This is the meaning of death: the ultimate self-dedication to the divine. Death so understood will not be distorted by the craving for immortality, for this act of giving away is reciprocity, man's part for God's gift of life. For the pious man it is a privilege to die."

Each one of us, from the time of our birth has, embedded in our minds and hearts, the choice of being able to do good or evil, be strong or weak, and to change the course of our lives and achieve a high level of happiness.

The choices that we make will determine whether, when we reach our final years, we will just give up and quietly await our last breath, live out our final years in anger over the process of aging, or, despite our physical, mental, and past experiences seek (as my cousin Ruth at age ninety-six has done) enjoyment from every moment of existence.

In his bestselling book, *Tuesdays With Morrie*, the well-known sports commentator and author, Mitch Alborn, tells the story of his relationship with his former teacher and friend Morrie Schwartz, and how, after learning that Morrie had ALS (Lou Gehrig's Disease), he began to visit with him each Tuesday and help Morrie through his final days.

The following is one example of how I lived that very experience many times in my lifetime:

Carl was a retired insurance representative who, at the age of sixty-five, was diagnosed with terminal lung cancer. He was divorced and had two children who did not live close to his small home in Las Vegas.

He contacted the Nathan Adelson Hospice asking for help, and I was assigned to provide him with friendship and some social activities so that he could live as reasonable a life as possible during his final years of life.

We met once or twice a week for three hours and did everything from discussing world issues to sharing meals to playing Gin Rummy, Checkers, Cribbage, etc.

He beat me at all of these games, which was most frustrating to me. In fact, one time after a really bad beating in a Cribbage game, I said to him, "If you were not dying, I would kill you."

We both had a hearty laugh.

Carl had a very large double bed and if he were not feeling well during a visit we would lie on it and discuss numerous subjects. On the night Ronald Reagan was elected President, we watched the unfolding event on television and voiced our political opinions.

Everything that brought me to the Clark County Morgue at the time of the previously mentioned MGM Fire on the night of November 22, 1980, and all that has happened since is exemplified by this event.

Nothing you have read in this book better summarizes why it is so important that the issues that have been raised be addressed not near or at the end of life's journey, but early on in the process.

I urge you, reader: No matter where you are on the road of life, stop and take inventory of who you really are and how you can begin to live every day of your life as if it were the last. In the final analysis, we are given the choice of living until we die or of accepting death before we die.

> "A man should hear a little music, read a little poetry, and see a fine picture every day of his life, in order that worldly cares may not obliterate the sense of the beautiful which God has implanted in the human soul."

—Johann Wolfgang von Goethe

SENIOR MOMENT #25

KNOWING YOUR MEANING OF LIFE CONTRIBUTES TO A HAPPY JOURNEY - PART DEUX

For many years, I was conflicted and trying to find the answer as to if there was, in fact, a thing (or person) called God, who predetermined all aspects of life. Bad things such as earthquakes, floods, wars, and accidents, and if God predetermined happy things as well, like weddings, births, successes in education, business, etc.

As I traveled life's road I began to understand—as will you—that it was planned to be that way. While nature and God play in role in life's cycle, we as individuals can do much to lessen the affects of the bad things and gain much from the joy of life.

For those who do not believe in God, or a higher power, please replace the word with this: "The Inexplicable."

Although it has been made very clear, in earlier chapters, that this book is not about religion and that I respect all creeds, by the same token, to deny that as we all go through life, our faith (or even spirituality) does not influence our thinking would be avoiding reality.

How many times a day do we hear the words, "I am praying for you," "May God be with you," or "God is with you?" These are not just expressions to help sooth you during difficult times, but sincere beliefs of those who know you, and even strangers who may, through a conversation with you or a family member, learn of the sadness with which you are dealing.

Almost daily we hear reports that fewer and fewer people are attending religious services, but does that really indicate that people do not have faith? I would suggest that we need to separate spirituality and faith from religious practice. Reading prayers and observing our religious practices is one thing; believing the teachings of our religion is quite another.

We need to understand that at the same time that mankind is seeking the help/guidance of God, God is seeking the love and support of mankind. The biblical story of Jacob's Ladder demonstrates that faith and spirituality comes from our reaching for the heavens. The strength to move through the dark days of life comes from the heavens extending its love and support to us.

Human beings are part of God and nature's world. Science has pretty much proven that while proper diet and exercise may be a major factor in how well the body does through the journey, we also know that our mental state can be greatly influenced by how we use our spirituality and faith.

During a lecture given to a group of senior citizens, a well-known psychologist gave a quotation which basically said that aging is determined by the mount of stress we had.

This shocked me. When I asked if that meant that if we had no stress we would not age, he quickly backed down. Aging is natural, but how we age can be certainly be affected by stress.

How can we make a difference in our destiny? By living a life at peace with ourselves, our family and community, finding happiness in each day through the way we live our lives, and finding our faith and spirituality to support us during both happy and difficult times.

Unless we understand that there is a purpose to life, almost all human beings seek the strength to overcome the difficulties that life sometimes puts in the path of our journey. This is, possibly, as a test of our durability.

Perhaps that is what is meant by the expression, "Looking up to the mountaintop and having faith, through our spiritual strength, that tomorrow will be a better day than today."

Even those amongst us who do not regularly attend "religious" services at the church of our choice turn to prayer at times of stress and illness. So let us look at this issue and see how does help us heal.

Why would we do that if we did not ultimately realize that there is a presence of God which we turn to for the strength? In order to be strong, we need to realize that God is at the same time really looking to us to demonstrate our ability to make this a better world.

Mildred is a seventy-year-old widow and is very lonely. She decides
to get a parrot as a companion to bring some activity to her home.
She goes to the neighborhood pet shop and finds a beautiful bird, but
it keeps singing out, "My name is Thelma and I am a hooker."

The pet shop owner assures her that this will stop once she gets the
bird home and starts speaking to her. So, she takes the bird home,
but it keeps singing out, "My name is Thelma and I am a hooker."

Mildred goes to her minister and asks his advice, as she is
embarrassed by the parrot's constant singing out of that phrase.

The minister is sympathetic and tells Mildred to bring the parrot to the
church, where he has his own parrot, who he tells her does nothing but sit
on the bottom rung of his cage and pray. He tells Mildred that by putting
her parrot in the cage with his, his parrot will get hers straightened out.

Mildred brings her parrot to the church. They put her parrot
on the top rung of the cage and leave the room.

Mildred's parrot sings out, "My name is Thelma and I am
a hooker." The minister's parrot stops praying, looks up at
Mildred's and sings out, "My prayers have been answered!"

In essence, we are doing two things we pray:

1. Reaching out and asking our faith to give us the strength to heal us and/or those who we are praying for.

2. Speaking to our deep spirituality in order to gather the strength to be able to deal with the events that are unfolding, and acknowledging that while we may not be able to control the outcome, we do have the capability of coming through our ordeal with resolve.

I saw how this process, while it did not have the positive results that I would have liked to have achieved, worked during Anna's illness. She was not a deeply religious person, but she did believe that there was God within her, as do I. For three years each day, we called upon our inner souls to help us deal with her challenges and keep a strong positive attitude.

My friend Mimi, Anna's caregiver, commented to me some six months after Anna's passing that in all of her caregiving experience she had never seen two people, Anna and myself, who never complained about what was happening and always had a confident attitude that we would get through the storm and move on to a peaceful new world for her and a renewed faith in life for me.

Praying, sadness, weeping, and laughter are all part of what might be considered the therapy of life. Consider this: If we had not had been given the ability to speak, we could not openly pray. Had not we been given the ability to shed tears, we not have the ability to cry or laugh.

A poet wrote, "If the eyes have no tears, the soul will have no rainbows." Our Faith calls for us to understand that challenges are part of life and that we need to use all of the tools we are provided with—our beliefs, physical capabilities, and mental strength—to get through the difficult times we often encounter as we travel life's pathway.

Yes, spirituality and faith play a major role in that process, so long as we understand that they are not always capable of providing the result we desire. However, they are there helping us to emerge from the crisis and also to achieve our objectives.

In an earlier chapter, I referred to the fourth element of life as being "hope" in the final analysis that is what we look to through our prayers.

> "He has seen but half of the universe who has
> never been shown the house of pain."

—Emerson

Welcome to the home of the human being.

SENIOR MOMENT #26

MEDITATION AND MINDFULLNESS CAN MAKE LIFE'S JOURNEY MORE SATISFYING

Certainly, we can all agree that while advances in medical science have, and continue, to help find cures for many diseases, and even prolong life—even when the challenges that some individuals endure as a result may not be worth the cure—it is also true that there are often things that we can individually do to help ourselves.

The practice of meditation and mindfulness, which were introduced by Buddhism, have become very important self-help methods which allow us to deal with pain, depression, and a whole list of life's problems.

One of the great lessons that Anna taught me was the importance for all of us to stop, look within ourselves each day, and take stock at where we are in life.

This has nothing to do with religious philosophy, but rather, it is all about taking a deep breath and looking at ourselves and our world by "climbing the mountain" before moving on.

What this means is that we need to raise ourselves above the daily routine, isolate ourselves from the world, and look out into the vision of our lives and where we are, what we want to accomplish, and what we need to do to achieve our dream.

We may not find the answers right away, but being mindful of the need to do so allows us to move on with life and think about how we will get to our destination happily and with a sense of accomplishment.

The Transcendentalist William David Thoreau did that when he took two years and two months out of his life to spend alone at Walden Pond. Recently, NBC announced that Johns Hopkins had done a major study on meditation and reported that it was extremely beneficial to those who learned how to practice it.

This is not to suggest that we can all afford to withdraw from our daily activities for such an extended period of time, but we can, however, spend thirty minutes each day in solitary retreat to refresh our minds and hearts.

> "I went to the woods because I wished to live deliberately, to
> front only the essential facts of life, and see if I could not learn
> what it had to teach, and not, when I came to die, discover that
> I had not lived. I did not wish to live what was not life..."

—Henry David Thoreau, *Walden Park*

How wonderful our journey could be if only we, like Thoreau, would take time each day to rediscover ourselves.

Do you agree?

So take a deep breath as we approach the end of our journey, and let's see how meditation can add joy to life's journey.

> "If I can't do anything useful, at least I would at
> least like to do as little harm as possible."

—Abisma

Now certainly no one can claim that meditation is a simple, or even a major factor in such situations, but it does work for many individuals and is certainly worthy of including it in our daily activities.

Far too many persons look upon meditation and mindfulness as cultish or religious methodology and thus deny themselves the opportunity to enrich their lives by removing much of the burdens they carry with themselves each day.

Ask yourself this question: "If by spending a minimum of fifteen to thirty minutes by myself each day, I could reinvent myself, become relaxed, see my life as it really is, and enjoy the rest of the journey free of all of the anxieties I live with, would I find that time?

What wise person would refuse to do so?

The author and poet Jon Kabat Zinn, in his well-known book on meditation and mindfulness, explains, "It is possible through meditation to find shelter from much of the wind that agitates the mind. Over time, a good deal of the turbulence may die down from lack of continuous feeding. But ultimately the winds of life and of the mind will blow, do what we may. Meditation is about knowing something about this and how to work with it."

Given the fast pace of our daily lives, it is no wonder that so many individuals feel tired and mentally, physically, and psychologically challenged as they travel life's pathway. Taking a pause to clear the mind and evaluate where you have been, where you are, and where you are going can make a major difference in where you end up and when.

That is what mediation is about. Being mindful of your circumstances and being able with a clear mind to make decisions about how to deal with today's wants, as well as tomorrows goals and allows us to become the person we really are and not the one that peer pressure often leads us to be who we are not.

> "Not to have pain is not to have been human."
>
> —Yiddish Proverb

As I was growing up I always enjoyed watching my mother and her mother, who lived with us, cook and bake up a storm. After all, isn't that what good Jewish woman did? (Ha-ha.) And of course, while we were never allowed in the kitchen to help, we did get to "eat the crumbs."

Eventually, I was married and began to fool around in the kitchen (cooking, that is). And then through some miracle of life I found a career in the food and beverage industry, took to it like a fish takes to water, and became what my friends who never want to go out to dinner, but prefer to eat my goodies, called a "great cook."

During that process I discovered the adjunct to meditation and meaningful mindfulness—the ability to look at life that was happening all around me, as well as my own activities while cooking almost automatically at the same time. In fact, as I was writing this book, I was writing and coming up with ideas for it as I cooked. I was then quickly going to the computer to put those thoughts down as the cooking process proceeded.

And while I found that to happen easily, it may take others some time to master the technique, but what a wonderful way to contemplate our daily activities, shopping, cooking, cleaning the house, etc.

Meditation techniques vary, but whether you do it sitting down, standing, or walking, it's no matter. All that matters is that you do so by understanding that the purpose is not to analyze and think about a particular issue you are dealing with, but the most rewarding purpose, instead, is clearing your mind of all that is going on in your life and look at your inner self each day.

> "You can't stop the waves, but you can learn to surf."

> —Swami Satchitananda

If you do nothing else but remember the Ahimsa, which is quoted at the start of this chapter, and examine your inner-self through the meditation mindfulness practice, you will be on your way to relieving your mind of some of the burdens you carry with you each day.

> "If you can't love King George V, or say Sir Winston Churchill,
> start with your wife, or your husband, or your children. Try to
> put their welfare first and your own last every minute of the day,
> and let the circle of your love expand from there. As long as you
> are trying your best, there can be no question of failure."

> —Mahatma Ghandi

Regardless of your age, health, or station in life, take a deep breath, stop all of life's actions, and take a hard look at yourself with an open mind. Be willing to make the changes needed in order not be hard on your body and soul, and not do things to harm others, and you will finally find a path that is meaningful.

How sad it is that we have allowed our society to become so fast tracked that most people are almost robot-like in their daily living? They don't take the time to step back and really look at their inner selves and ask, "Who am I? Where am I? Where am I headed?"

It is like the efficiency expert who was speaking to a group of people on the topic of why it is important to carefully prepare and plan your life on what you are considering, what you are going to do, and all the possible consequences of your proposed actions.

He gave the class an example: "I studied my wife's breakfast routine for many years. She made multiple trips between the refrigerator, the kitchen counter, the stove, the pantry, and the dishwasher, usually carrying one item at a time.

A person in the audience asked, "And did it save time?"

To which the expert said, "Yes, it did. It used to take her twenty-five minutes to make breakfast; now I do it in nine minutes."

How much easier and relaxed our journey could be if only we would take time each day to rediscover ourselves.

A Note to My Readers

I confess that I have no idea what the source of the following story is, but it seems to me it fits quite well into the fun we can have as we journey through life by laughing at ourselves. It is a letter that was supposedly sent to Ann Landers some year ago.

Dear Ann,

Over the years I have had a great deal of pleasure from your column, and as a physician, I commend you for the fine job you do in the health field.

Here is something that a friend sent me in the mail recently. I don't know who wrote it, but it gave me the best laugh I've had in a long time. I hope you will share it with your readers.

Your Friend,

(Name omitted for ethical reasons)

⇒◆⇐

Dear-------,

I agree. It's a hoot. What a way to start the week. Thanks for sending it my way.

What Not To Name Your Dog

Everybody who has a dog calls him "Rover" or "Boy." I call mine "Sex." He's a great pal, but he has caused me a great deal of embarrassment.

When I went to city hall to renew his dog license, I told the clerk I would like a license for Sex. He said, "I would like one too!" Then I said, "But this is a dog." He said he didn't care what she looked like. Then I said, "You don't understand. I have had Sex since I was nine years old." He winked and said, "You must have been quite a kid."

When I got married and went on my honeymoon, I took the dog with me. I told the motel clerk that I wanted a room for my wife and me, and a special room for Sex.

He said, "You don't need a special room. As long as you pay your bill, we don't care what you do."

I said, "Look, you don't seem to understand. Sex keeps me awake at night." The clerk said. "Funny, I have the same problem."

One day I entered Sex in a contest, but before the competition began, the dog ran away. Another contestant asked me why I was just standing there looking disappointed. I told him I had planned to have Sex in the contest.

He told me I should have sold my own tickets. "But you don't understand," I said. "I had hoped to have Sex on TV."

He said, "Now that cable is all over the place, it's no big deal anymore."

When my wife and I separated, we went to court to fight for custody of the dog. I said, "Your Honor, I had Sex before I was married." The judge said, "This court is not a confessional. Stick to the case, please."

Then I told him that after I was married, Sex left me. He said, "Me too."

Last night, Sex ran off again. I spent hours looking around town for him. A cop came by and asked, "What are you doing in this alley at four o'clock in the morning?"

I told him I was looking for Sex.

My case comes up on Friday.

SENIOR MOMENT #27

DON'T LET TECHNOLOGY CONTROL YOUR LIFE

"There's nothing like a newborn baby to
renew your spirit—and to buttress your
resolve to make the world a better place."

—Virginia Kelley (1923–1994)

Technology and scientific advances have made a dramatic impact on humanity, both positive and negative. And while we are all keenly aware of the positive aspects of these accomplishments, what we fail to recognize and adapt to are the negatives and how they affect us throughout as we approach our inevitable arrival at out final destination.

Join with me and observe, as I have, the impact of how technology has diminished one of the most important elements of life: the role of the father and mother as the primary teachers of our children.

You need only talk to school teachers and they will tell you that getting the parents of their students to be involved in their child's education is one of their most difficult tasks.

There was a time when parents in my generation spent a major part of their time with their children: on weekends, after school, and whenever the youngsters had free time.

School was the place we sent children to receive knowledge about things, events, places, history, etc. At night we sat around the dinner table and discussed what we had learned that day and how it applied to our lives.

This allowed our parents to speak to their children, explain and expand on what they had learned, and have discussions about life and its consequences with their family members.

In effect, parents were advanced educators of their kids and influenced their character and actions while preparing them for life. Today, parents thrive on being their child's friend and not on being their guide through life.

Today, Dad is busy driving the freeways from early morning to night, wrapped up in meetings that will help finance a lifestyle or just pay the bills, and out playing golf with business associates.

Mom is either working long hours, finding ways to keep the kids occupied so that she is free to do her thing, and the children are left to watch TV, fool around on the computer, or spend their time—even when sitting and having dinner with the family—talking to friends on their iPhone. They are often left with babysitters to ensure that someone is with them.

And on top of all of that, our education system has gone the route of eliminating homework, as well as doing away with books. Instead, they just use tablets and other scaled-down resources.

Those of us who grew up during the Great Depression can well remember the following wise words: "Everything you ever wanted to know can be found in a book."

Technology may well serve many of our needs, but to me, the fact that people are slowly replacing the books on their bookshelves with iPads removes one of the most valuable sources of learning about life. How many persons really go back to the computer once they have quickly read a book, and how do our children learn when there is no bookshelf filled with knowledge to excite their curiosity?

> "Although I'm only fourteen, I know quite well what I want. I know who is right and who is wrong. I have my opinions, my own ideas and principles, and although it may sound pretty mad from an adolescent, I feel more of a person than a child, I feel quite independent of anyone."

> —**_Anne Frank_**, _The Diary of Anne Frank_

In fact, in many homes there is no "family dinner." Everyone is busy running around, going out, taking dance lessons, playing soccer, and being involved in activities that may bring parents bragging rights, but do nothing to really enrich their children or prepare them for the real issues of life.

The youth of today have no real role models to help shape their lives, and this sad reality has led to increased cultist involvement, drug and alcohol abuse, and all sorts of other social issues.

Who is the teacher of our youth? How can we expect them to develop emotionally, intellectually, and yes, maturely if their teachers—their parents—are themselves not good role models?

A father came home late after a long day at work and was sitting and reading his newspaper with his ten-year-old son next to him. The son asked, "Dad, how do we know that the world is round?"

The father, while continuing to read his paper grunted, "I don't know!"

The son then asked his dad, "What makes the sun and moon change places?"

Again, the father grunted, "I don't know."

The son says, "Dad, I'm sorry for asking such dumb questions." The father replies, "That's okay, son. If you don't ask questions you will never learn anything."

If we are to make a better world, we need to, by example, demonstrate to our youth that life is not about being rewarded by our parents for doing what they want us to do while setting bad examples for them by failing to be good teachers. It is equally important that we take the time to listen to and encourage them to follow a path that meets their own objectives in life.

More and more we judge our youth on their athletic agility, school grades, and other accomplishments and not on their ability to think and have a vision of life that differs from their parents' vision for them.

If you want to get a real eye opener, sit down and talk with a teenager. Ask them what they think about life and what they really are interested in doing. I actually did that in writing this chapter and was amazed to hear such statements as:

"My dad says I should try to make the football team," and "My mom told me that she would really, really love me if I got a scholarship to college."

Did anyone ever ask these children what would make them happy, or for that matter, introduce them to the kinds of things they should consider when thinking about their future?

And consider this: While parents go out of their way to shield youth from the dark side of life, they, in a way, prevent them from seeing the joy and happiness that awaits them. If they understand life's challenges, even at the youngest age, our children should hear about such matters. They understand what is going on around them better than we think.

Let me share with you one of the most interesting and humorous true stories that so eloquently makes this point. It actually happened, and involved my great-grandson, Tripp:

Tripp's mother was preparing for the arrival of a new baby and his parents were moving to a new home in anticipation of a larger family.

Because of this, they had put some of their living room furniture up for sale and had made arrangements for a buyer to pick it up. My granddaughter, Jennifer, called her mother and asked her to pick Tripp up at his preschool and bring him home so that she could complete the sale.

When Judi, her mother, brought Tripp home, he sat down on the only piece of furniture left in the room: the coffee table. Jennifer asked him if he saw anything different about their living room, as it was obviously pretty empty. Tripp said no.

Again, she asked him if he had noticed anything unusual, particularly the spaces where the furniture had stood.

He looked at her and said, "Why do you think I am sitting on the table?"

Never assume that the young are not aware of what is going on around them, and be certain to explain the ways of life, good and bad.

———⋙•⋘———

A seven-year-old girl runs out to her backyard and asks her
father, who is doing some gardening, "Daddy, what is sex?

The father is startled by the question, but sits down next to
her and discusses the birds and bees. He explains sexual
intercourse and conception. Tells her about sperm and
eggs, puberty, menstruation, men, women, love, etc.

He figures that is best to be truthful when his child asks
a question. The child, of course, is overwhelmed with all
of this new information she receives about life.

The father then asks her, "Why did you want me to tell you
all about sex?" to which she answers, "Because Mom just
told me that lunch would be ready in a few secs."

———⋙•⋘———

I have this message for all youth who are just beginning to merge onto the highway of life:
It is your life to live, and even though you will at first need the financial support of others,
live it as you see the highway. Seek advice, weigh it carefully, and then move along to
achieve *your* objectives, not somebody else's.

Remember that at life's end, you will carry the burden of its success—or failure. You cannot put the blame of failure on others.

"We get our parents when they are so old that
it is hard to change their habits."

And to all of the parents: Love your children for who they are; not for what you expect
them to be. Talk to and listen to them. I know my own life has been enriched by listening to
and watching my children and grandchildren do their thing—even when I might not have
done it their way.

There is one other element of family that has dramatically changed that has affected the life and attitude of our youth. There was a time when one or both grandparents lived with us, or very close by and greatly influenced us.

Today they live a long distance away or in a facility of one kind or another, and we see them mostly on special occasions. The wisdom of the aged is sadly missed in the lives of our children.

In his wonderful book *In God's Mirror,* Rabbi Harold Schulweis, my late friend (he passed away on December 18, 2014) and mentor writes:

> "When parents will not allow children to visit the sick relative
> in the hospital (except when health vulnerability is a factor)
> or attend the funeral of their grandmother lest they see human
> beings cry or mourn their loss, they rob them of their humanity,
> and prepare for the perpetual search for painkillers.

Their character is spoiled by parental over protection that reduces life to the avoidance of unpleasantness and the pursuit of proximate pleasure."

In reality, the Rabbi suggests that we too often choose pleasure when we should pursue life.

Parents who would deny the youth in their lives the right to know or feel all of the emotions of life are, in effect, denying them the ability to understand the real meaning of life until it's too late.

> "The first half of our life is ruined by our parents;
> the second half by our children."

> —Clarence Darrow

Let me share two examples of how the parents of two well-known individuals affected the future of these two persons:

Jason, a very intelligent young man in his mid teens, was told by his parents that they wanted him to become a medical scientist and follow in the steps of other family members.

Jason really had no interest in doing that, but the parents told him that they would not support him financially or pay for his college education unless he did so. And thus he, being an all "A" student, was easily admitted to the professional school of their choice. After one semester, he knew he had made a mistake, and so he deliberately failed his final exams and was asked to leave that school.

He then went to a different specialty; one that he had told his parents was what he wanted to do. He completed a four-year course in three years and has gone on to be one of the most recognized and highest-paid executives in his chosen career, much to the disappointment of his family.

"Don't limit a child to *your* own learning,
for he was born in another time."

Alice, a seventeen year old, was a vivaciously popular student who had a 3.5 grade point average as she went through elementary, middle, and high school. She was very popular with her fellow students and seemed destined for big things as she approached college age.

Her parents insisted that they would not pay for her education unless she pursued a degree in Psychology. Surprisingly, her high school counselor had told her parents that she was not good college material.

After two years of pursuing her degree, she decided that school was not for her. She quit and found a menial job in the business world. Her parents were most upset. Undeterred, Alice took some business courses at night and has gone on to be a top executive in a major corporation.

We need to always encourage our youth to follow their dream and not ours, while at the same time being there to listen, guide, and help them as they move on to the various stages of life.

———◇———

"A doctor was very busy working in his study when his small son
came into the room and stood silently watching him. The doctor was
preoccupied with his work. He put his hand in his pocket took out a coin
and handed it to the child. "I don't want any money," the boy said.

The doctor then opened a drawer of his desk, took out a candy
bar, and offered it to his son. Again, the boy refused the offer.

The doctor was very impatient and very busy, so he
asked his son, "What is it that you want?

"I don't want anything, replied the son. "I just wanted to be with you."

The youth of today will be our caregivers of tomorrow. We need to be certain not only that they are prepared to fill that role, but that we show them the way.

One need only visit the care centers which house our elderly to really understand how what we do when they are in their formative years shapes their thinking and attitude about our second dchildhood."

And suddenly we are past the stage of youth where we have hopefully gained the wisdom to know who we are and where we are headed. We move on to middle age, and a whole new set of issues confronts us.

Our parents and siblings have taken on new roles, and we have watched as our grandparents and other relatives have aged. Soon our youth is gone and we will assume the awesome dual roles of teachers of our children and caregivers of our parents.

Unless we begin—along with all of those around us—to prepare for this great task, suddenly being confronted with it can create a major crisis in our lives, as well as all others involved.

"They who educate children well are more to be honored than those who
produce them: for these only gave them life, they the art of living."

—Aristotle

As we move on receive our education and/or begin to implement our chosen career path, find our love, and possibly begin to raise a family, we move into the middle part of our lives. We both see and feel the results of decisions we have made as we experience the effects of life, both good and bad.

And think about this: When you begin to start a family, what you are about to do is give birth to your future caregivers. From this point forward, family relationships become even more critical.

"I love my parents. They're wonderful people, but they were very strict, and I still look for ways to get even. When I got my own apartment for the very first time and they came to stay with me for the weekend, I made them stay in separate bedrooms."

—Elaine Bernstein Partnow

Middle age is that time of life when we think about career changes, where we have been, and where we would like to go. As Victor Frankl points out in his exciting book *Man's Search for Meaning,* "It is not always what man can teach life, but what life can teach us."

There are all kinds of case studies about mid-life crises. They tell the sad story of what happens when we, both men and women, realize that we are stuck in a career we don't like, a marriage which we see as not being meaningful, and a lifestyle which does not blend with our vision of life.

We are afraid to lose our income, fearful of the breakup of our family, and not wanting to disappoint our loved ones. We drift to a place in life where we begin to do things that are not in our character. Far too many are turning to secret lives, drugs, alcohol, suicide, etc.

There is a growing pressure on all families to become more involved mentally, physically, and financially with the care of their parents and other close family members who are aging. The financial and time burden this is imposing on society is a fast-growing problem for all of us.

Middle age is also about the time that the kinds of things like resentments, divorces, jealousies, religious and political differences, and financial conflicts begin to tear families apart rather bring them together.

And so just as at a time when we are moving towards the final phase of life—which for some it will be earlier than others—we are letting petty difference drive a wedge between us.

"This world would be for us a happier place
And there would be less regretting

If we could remember to practice with grace
The very fine art of forgetting."

—Morris Mandel, *Stories for Speakers*

At this critical time in our lives, we need to stop and take inventory of who we are, where we are in life, and where we want to go. The following story is an incredibly story about a very busty person who explained what this phase of our lives would look like if only we would practice mindfulness while being involved in our daily tasks.

"Something wonderful happened to me the other night. I really lucked out. Everyone should be so lucky. I had no business to take care of, no meetings to attend, and no social arrangements to keep, so I stayed home.

What a fantastic experience it was. I got to play with the kids, watch television with the entire family, spend time talking and cuddling with my wife, read the newspaper, and just relax.

How exciting! I think I will join the organization called "Stay at Home."

⊰•⊱

It is in this phase of life that we need to make certain that we have brought our family to-gether to talk about our thoughts about "tomorrow," make our plans for the remainder of our life, and realistically prepare not only for our retirement, but for the final stretch of the journey.

> "Shortly after an elderly, white-haired woman visitor left their home,
> a young girl said to her mother, 'If I could be such a beautiful, sweet,
> loveable person, I would not fear getting old.' The mother replied, 'If you
> really want to be that kind of old woman, you had better start now. She
> does not seem to me to be the kind of work that was done in a hurry."

Slowly but surely, we reach the final phase of our lives, when our children are either off to school, getting into their careers, married, and often no longer living at home. Some are even starting their own families.

At the same time, we may be beginning to have some health issues, thinking about retire-ment, or suddenly having to face the reality of having to care for our parents who have or are near the end of their journey.

I spoke to the son-in-law of a friend in his late sixties who had recently lost his wife to a sudden illness. She was in her early sixties. He told me that he had pleaded with his in-laws for several years to make plans for their aging process, but that they had refused, saying it was not time.

He finally convinced them to do so shortly before she became ill. He told me how his father-in-law had thanked him for having the foresight to get them to act and how much easier that had made it for the entire family.

When you chose life, it also includes death, and it needs to be looked at as such. If we openly accept that fact, do what we "have" to do to prepare for it, and go on living our lives to the full extent of happiness, what better way to enjoy the fruits of our labor.

———⊱⋅⊰———

The holidays were approaching, and an elderly mother who lived in a home for the aged some distance from her middle-age son responded to the delivery of some flowers she received from him with the following letter:

"To my precious son and the woman who he mistakenly decided to marry,

Happy Holidays,

Thank you for the lovely flowers, which I have carefully wrapped and frozen so that they are ready for my grave. Please do not worry about me. While I am having great difficulty breathing, I am doing pretty well. What is more important is that all of you enjoy the holidays even though you live such a distance from your very sick mother.

Included with this letter are my last few dollars which, hopefully, you will use to buy gifts for my grandchildren, which your wife would most certainly never otherwise do.

By the way, while I know that Grandma died some year ago, she never really had a decent funeral, so Aunt Shirley and I dug her up and reburied her last week. I knew that that person you married would not let you attend the service, so I did not invite you. She probably didn't even show you the video I sent of my recent abdominal surgery.

The time has come for me to sign off and get to sleep. It takes me a while to get into the bedroom because I lost my cane a few days ago trying to avoid some muggers. Also, I have to find some additional blankets because my heat was turned off last week.

I know how important your long, expensive holiday vacations are to you and that woman, so please do not spend any more money on me.

Please give my grandchildren a big kiss for me and my regards to that person—whoever she is—who took you away from my life."

I love you,

Mother

—Anonymous

Obviously this letter was included herein in jest, but sadly, as I have witnessed every day since researching this document, it is filled with truism. If those who are just entering adulthood observe this kind of anger and bitterness coming from those who they are following, it's hard not to come away with a distorted view of life.

The lesson to be learned from all of this is that from the time we are born and reach start of adulthood, we are observing life and digesting the events that we see taking place in the lives of our parents.

If they do not answer our unspoken questions about what the meaning is of all that is taking place before our eyes and explain the events as they occur, we are left to figure out the answers as we travel the journey.

As reach middle age and are beginning to become responsible for the decisions that were once made by our parents, we are faced with the ordeal of trying to understand what happened and what to do about it.

And by that time, our parents really need our help because they did not prepare themselves or us for the aging process. How much better would our lives be if we were well prepared early on?

> "Remember an expert was once a beginner. The earlier you begin, the sooner you will have the expertise to handle life's challenges."

"The first half of our life is ruined by our parents;
the second half by our children."

—Clarence Darrow

We've spent a great deal of time together. Birth to the end of life. Let's not say "death" anymore. Who knows what happens after? Let's simply say, "End of life."

A few random thoughts as I wrap up:

Nothing can replace humanity. What do I mean by that? Technology, machines—we can utilize it all, everything we have developed, but nothing can take the place of the love and kindness of another human being during this journey we call "life."

Nor can machines plan for you, by the way.

Technology can replace neither parents, family, friends, nor teachers. Computers, cell phones, and other technology have their place, but they are not, nor can they be, replacements. Remember this, as it's far too easy to let machines "do the job."

Big mistake.

Those of us who grew up during the Great Depression, well before the advent of all our modern tech, can well remember the following wise words: "Everything you ever wanted to know can be found in a book."

That being said, neither does a book replace the human. Remember this too.

Today, as an example of what technology "lacks," there is no longer a family dinner in many homes. The source of some of our greatest information and wisdom through the ages, the family, has been replaced by computer tablets and phones that can do everything except give you a hug.

In my opinion, leaning exclusively on technology at the expense of humanity does nothing to really enrich their children or prepare them for the real issues of life.

Can an iPad help a child develop emotionally? I don't think so...

For a better life and a more fulfilling journey, regularly ask your children what makes them happy, and then work their answers into a guided method of introducing them to the kinds of things they should consider when thinking about their future.

The type of information I have included in this book.

Kids believe they are immortal, but trust me, they rarely think about a future because they are not always taken seriously. Ask the right questions, guide them well, and by the end, your care, preparation, and humanity will aid them immensely in the difficult road that is called "life" and "end of life."

And thus, the wisdom of the aged becomes an everlasting force, as your children will pass your teachings onto your children's children and so on.

And the world becomes a better place.

Thank you, everyone. I appreciate the indulgence.

Until we meet again, I leave you with the following heartfelt message: May you live your life every day sharing your love with all you know.

SENIOR MOMENT #29

DECISIONS WE MAKE CAN AFFECT OUR HAPPINESS

*"An idealist is one who, on noticing that a rose smells better than
a cabbage, concluded that it will also make a better soup."*

—H. L. Menchen

From our earliest days until the end of life, we have been given the task of making decisions that not only involve our own life, but also the lives of others.

Regardless of whether they involve our daily activities, choosing a career path, health issues, the aging process of those we love, or our own, it is most important that we form a concept in our minds about how we are going to make the choices we have and what questions we need to consider in making them.

Many of these decisions also involve our view of morality and right and wrong. Sometimes, for example, your moral values may say that this is the wrong decision, but by society's values, it is the right one.

I spoke to an elderly man who told me that early in his life he was faced with a family crisis, and he had to make a choice between doing something which clearly violated his sense of moral values or saving the cohesiveness of his family.

He chose to save his family and will carry the shame of his actions to his grave rather than hurt his family by revealing all of the factors which led him to make the choice he did.

Sometimes we make choices without seeking advice because we are afraid the advice will prevent us from doing what we have already made up our minds to do. In fact, in my work as a consultant to major business enterprises, before I begin the project or make recommendations the first question I ask my client is, "Have you already make up your mind about what you want to do? If they say yes, I turn down the work. Why waste my time?

———◆———

A middle-aged schoolteacher who invested her life's savings in a business enterprise which had been elaborately explained to her by a swindler.

When her investment disappeared and the wonderful dream was shattered, she went to the office of the Better Business Bureau. "Why on Earth," they asked her, "didn't you come to us first? Didn't you know about the Better Business Bureau?"

"Oh yes," said the lady, sadly. "I've always known about you, but I didn't come to you because I was afraid you'd tell me not to do it."

—Bits and Pieces

———◆———

One of my favorite writers is Frank Bures. His articles appear regularly in many publications, including the Rotarian. In the December 2013 issue, he writes about how important is it to "aspire to high principles," but not to go overboard.

In speaking about his companion, Bridget, Bures writes that she believes that living a good life means striking a balance between the causes you believe in and the people you loved; between the world and your home; between your ideals and your community.

All decisions you make should take this concept into consideration. As we travel life's road we need to understand that the most important decisions we are called upon to make have nothing to do with the issues I raised earlier in this chapter, and everything to do with our future, our relationships with family and friends, and our destiny as we go through life.

Rarely do they require immediate finality, but there is reasonable time to make them. However, one must start early in life to define them, plan them, and implement them.

What we do not have is twenty-four hour notice to put them into place. And if we do begin the process early and plan the predictable decisions then we will be better prepared and ready when we are faced with making the inevitable uninvited, unanticipated, unavoidable decisions which come to us like a snowball out of Hell.

One of the lessons that I have learned over my lifetime is that when decision-making issues over which I have control are presented to me by others, they require a fast answer.

And if I am hesitant in anyway, I will say no as a first response and then take some time to mull over the issue. Later, if I see its merits, I will change my mind and say yes.

Once you say yes, it is very difficult to justify saying no. And by the same token, if you realize you have made a very bad decision, do not be so proud that you cannot admit it and reverse your action.

I recall reading that historians have reported that when the final draft of the Emancipation Declaration was handed to Abraham Lincoln, his hands shook and he told his staff to bring it back the next day, as he was not comfortable signing it. After getting a good night's sleep and re-reading it, he signed it the following morning.

Earlier in this chapter I mentioned that in making decisions, you need to consider two important things: how it will affect others, and how it will affect you and your future. If it will be mostly beneficial to them, you may have to swallow hard and encourage them to move ahead.

Some years ago, while working on a major project for a large international corporation, I had the privilege of meeting, working with, and training a very beautiful, intelligent and single young woman. One day, she confided in me that she was pregnant and was considering an abortion.

I immediately advised her not to do so, but instead have the child and dedicate herself to raising it. When she asked me why, I told her that she was very smart and had a good future, but that she was living a wild life and needed to get herself under control. I told her that she would eventually find the right man and marry.

After thinking about it, she called me and told me she was going to follow my advice. She had the baby, went on to get a major college degree, and has been practicing a well-known profession for many years.

Her son is personable, handsome, and moving towards success in his field of work. The family is vibrant, filled with love for each other, and enjoying much success. We keep in touch and she always thanks me for my guidance when all I did was give her some common sense advice.

These are the kinds of decisions life's experiences are built on—decisions all of us has the ability to make so as to help others and ourselves enjoy life fully and completely.

I know of no better way to explain the point being made here about every decision we make has an effect on some on others than the words of Harry Emerson Fosdick, who wrote:

"We ask the leaf, 'Are you complete in yourself?' and the leaf answers, 'No, my life is in the branches.' We ask the branch and the branch answers, 'No, my life is in the root." Ask the root and it answers, 'No, my life is in the trunk and branches and leaves. Keep the branches stripped of leaves, and I shall die.'" Consider unexpected obstacles that stand in the way of decisions we think are good and sometimes bring us sadness.

⥼⬦⥽

A young man comes to his father and mother and tells them
that he is in love and is going to marry a very beautiful
girl. He tells them her name is Susan Brown.

The young man's father takes him aside and tells him that he cannot
marry Susan because when he and his wife married years ago, the
wife was not a good bed partner and so he, the father, had an affair
with another woman and that Susan Brown was the son's step sister.

The son was very upset, but started dating other women. Some months
later, he again came to his parents to announce that he had fallen in
love with Sherry Williams and that they were going to be married.

Once again, the father took him aside and repeated the
same story; only this time Sherry was his half sister.

The son could not conceal his anger and he went to
his mother and told her what had happened.

He told his mother that his father was killing any chance he had of
getting married. His mother told him not to pay any attention to what
the father said, because he really wasn't the son's real father.

SENIOR MOMENT #30

DO NOT LET PETTY ISSUES DESTROY PERSONAL RELATIONSHIPS

"There was a wise man who presented each of his children as they entered adulthood with a scale. When they asked him why, he told them that as they went through life they would encounter situations which tested their ability to deal with anger and forgiveness, and they would need to carefully balance their desire to punish those whom they thought had hurt them against the goodness that they inherently had and find a way to forgive and go on to a greater happiness."

—Bernie Otis

It would be natural to ask what the subjects of anger and forgiveness have to do with the journey through life and why it needs to be discussed as part of the Preparation for Old Age.

If you stop and think about it, some of the most painful periods of our lives revolve around these very issues. As I interviewed people of all ages for this book, the terms "dysfunctional,' 'bitter,' 'disruptive, 'hate,' etc. were commonly used in answer to my questions about family relationships, personal friendships, and business dealings.

And do not think for a moment that our children do not see and hear our reaction to such relationships and end up factoring our resentments into their future handling of similar circumstances.

One cannot read the stories told in the Old and New Testaments, as well as other historical documents about life through the ages, without recognizing that since the beginning of our existence the issues of anger and forgiveness have caused much distress to mankind. They have been a major factor in the breakup of families, as well as their reconciliation.

There is the story told of a young man who, while attending the fiftieth wedding anniversary of a family friend, jokingly asked the husband of the celebrants if during his long marriage he had ever considered divorce. The man quickly answered, "Divorce? Never. Murder? Numerous times."

It is one thing to express frustration in a humorous manner, it is quite another to shout angry words, act mean spirited, and carry this bitterness with us on a daily basis.

Henry asks his wife if she would like to go to Paris for her birthday. She tells him that does not interest her. "Well, how about a fur coat? He asks.

Again, she says it is not what she wants. "A diamond watch?" he suggests.

"No." she replies. "I was thinking about wanting a divorce." To which he replies, "I was not thinking of something that expensive."

How many times in your life has someone you know—family or friend—done something to you that clearly made you angry enough not to want them to be in your life?

Recently, I met a dear friend, eighty-five years of age. She told me that while engaged in a social card game with another woman her age, the other party realized she had no money. My friend loaned her fifty cents which the woman said she would pay back and never did.

My friend told me how angry she was at the other woman, and I asked her if it was worth getting herself so upset over such a ridiculous matter. She could not contain herself. I can never understand why we, as people, allow ourselves to end relationships and—even worse—impair our own well being. Especially over what, in almost all situations of anger, are so insignificant in the whole picture of life.

"Many people lose their tempers merely from seeing you keep yours."

—Frank Moore Kelly

There is a very active widower in his eighties who had just a few months earlier lost the woman he adored in their thirtieth year of marriage. While not actively seeking a new romance, he met a woman who completely captivated him.

In the process of advancing a relationship with her, he became overzealous because of jealousies and ill-conceived interpretations of this woman and others' relationship. He upset this beautiful woman to the point where she broke off the relationship and ceased speaking to him.

After taking some time to evaluate how important the relationship was to him and what he could have done differently to enhance it, he realized how very important she was to him and decide that the only way to try to rectify the situation was to take full responsibility for what had happened even though he sincerely believes that not all of the blame fell on him. That being said, it was not worth pointing fingers when what he desired was reconciliation.

In my lifetime I have seen the most incredible examples of true love lost, family breakups, and painful relationships taken to the grave over the unwillingness to reconcile differences. Many of these differences are over what, in the entire picture of life, are petty differences involving nothing more than hurt egos.

> "Learning to ignore things is one of the great paths to inner peace."

> —Anonymous

Sometimes when things go wrong in a relationship even if you are certain after careful thought that the other party was completely off base. By reflecting on how, in the scheme of things, being angry and upset will cause you long-term pain and end what should be an important relationship, moving on and enjoying life may be the better of solutions.

A father and son from a small European Country are visiting the
United States and are in a major shopping center. Their excitement
at all the things they see that are new to them is heightened by two
highly polished walls that move apart and come together again.

The young boy asks his father what they are and the father says he does
not know. Just then the walls separate and an elderly woman walks in

between them and the walls close. A few minutes later, the walls once again separate and a vivacious, beautiful young woman walks out.

The father is very quiet and then says to his son, "I really don't know what they are, but we need to get one for your mother."

"A vain man, a frightened man, bigoted man, or an angry man, cannot laugh at himself or be laughed at, but the man who can laugh at himself or be laughed at has taken another step towards the perfect sanity which brings peace on earth and good will to men."

—Credo of Nat Schmulowitz

SENIOR MOMENT #31

EARLY PREPARATION FOR THE TRIP'S END MAKES THE ARRIVAL THAT MUCH MORE ENJOYABLE

Consider this: When a family learns that they are going to have a new baby, what do they do immediately in the process is begin to purchase the:

- Crib
- Play pen
- High chair
- Car seat
- Bibs
- Diapers
- Misc. clothing
- Rocker
- Misc. items for feeding
- Blankets
- Assortment of other items necessary for to care for the expected child
- Some sort of minimal financial planning for their education

And once the child is born and it is an absolute given that eventually it will die, what is done over the years to prepare for that event? Practically nothing until an event happens to prompt a panic response in a limited time frame.

If only every human being could hear the horrors that occur in families all over the country because no advanced planning was done to prepare for this absolutely certain event, would it become so much easier.

In previous chapters of this book, I have made an effort to discuss the many issues of the journey through life and given many examples of events that could occur to both cause us pain and challenges and to help us have a happy, joyful life until the very end.

In this chapter you will find some of the questions you need to have the answers to long before the final destination is reached and, in fact, often occur quite unexpectedly early or midway through a normal life's journey.

As millions of individuals and families discover all to often procrastinating, or putting off asking the questions and documenting the answers just makes it that much more difficult to deal with when we are not ready.

While it is not possible any expert on this subject know every question to ask or what the correct answer in every individual's case is, the information provided in this chapter will certainly put you ahead of the game.

My own experience gained over the three years of my beloved's journey, plus my experience living in an assisted living center with persons and their families who have had hands-on experience makes me more than comfortable providing this information and knowing it is not theory, but fact.

In addition, I would strongly recommend that if an outside advocate or senior care advisor/professional is used to help you with this process that it is not enough that they are trained in their field of expertise, but it is absolutely essential that they have many detailed hands-on experiences dealing with individuals and families who have actually gone through the life/aging/death experience.

Just having a law, insurance, financial planning and/or license is not in itself insurance that you will get the best answers. (Please note that I have the highest respect for all professions.)

Finally, be certain to document all of the decisions and information herein discussed and have copies made and stored in an easy-to-find filing system/computer which is known to all of those involved in executing the plan.

A seventy-eight year old man went to his doctor because he was not feeling well. The doctor said he needed to get a sperm count and gave the man a jar to fill up telling him to bring it back the next day.

The next morning, he returned the jar to the doctor and it was empty. The doctor asked what happened and the man said he had a terrible time and could not do anything.

He said he tried with his right hand and then his left. He called his wife to help and she tried with her left hand, her right hand, and her mouth. Nothing. They called in the lady next door. The doctor said, "You did what?" and the man said she tried with her left hand and then her right, but they could not get the jar opened.

In other chapters of this book there was information and suggestions for the kinds of things individuals and families need to prepare for early in the journey of life.

The following is a list of the many other issues and questions that you need to ask in order to be as prepared as possible when the time comes to have the answers ready and action taken.

Keep in mind that those who will be primarily responsible for their loved ones' care must be ready and strong enough to not accept the wishes expressed by their love one. For example, while that person may express a desire to live alone at home, the ramifications of that could have disastrous effects.

Home and Personal Issues:

1. Do you have a list of all of your doctors and your relationship with them?

2. Do you have a list of your insurance plans, how to contact them, and how they are paid for?

3. Have we carefully gone through your home and evaluated it to be certain that the necessary safety conditions have been addressed?

4. In case of a home maintenance problem (plumbing, electrical, gardening, heating, etc.) who are to vendors that provide you with that service?

5. Do you have a home alert system in case you fall or need help, and how does it work?

6. I case the help of a neighbor is needed, who are the ones you are close with and how do we reach them?

7. Where in the home do you keep money, jewelry, and other valuable items?

8. Who is the insurer for those items mentioned in #7 and how do we reach them?

9. If you drive, where are the car keys kept, what insurance do you have, and how to we contact the insurer?

10. Is the car paid for, leased, etc. and who do we contact on those issues?

11. What credit obligations do you have, how do we contact the creditors, and where are the credit cards and documentation connected to them?

12. Who is going to be your primary caregiver and what authorization do they have to make decisions for you?

13. It would be natural to ask, " Why do I need to have answers to all of these questions? After all, I am young and my loved ones are just middle aged. We have time."

Unfortunately, things happen to young people as well as the middle aged, and to repeat what I have written elsewhere: Recent major studies have confirmed earlier ones that show at least twenty-five percent of aging illnesses like Alzheimer's begin around the age of fifty.

As I myself found out much too late, when you are most consumed with your own illness or the serious illness of loved ones, having to find the answers to these and the questions that follow is a burden far to heavy to bear.

Insurance and Care Giver Questions:

When it comes to caregivers, there are many additional issues that affect that subject. Let's take a look at them:

1. What kind of health, disability, long term, medication and other health policies are you covered by?

2. Do you have Medicare? Do you also have a supplemental health care policy that covers that portion of care that Medicare does not?

3. Are your credit cards and other financial assets protected by Credit Defense Programs?

4. Do your policies cover home health care programs?

5. Do you have list of contact information for all of the policies you have?

6. In the case where you are the primary recipient of the benefits and other family members are covered under that policy, what happens to their benefits if you pass away?

7. What are the waiting periods for activation of the pertinent policies?

8. Are your doctors aware of who to call in case there is a danger to your health?

9. What medications are you taking?

10. Do all of your doctors know what other physicians are caring for your various health issues?

It should be quite obvious when we look at the enormity of the issues involved in our preparation for the end of our journey, as well as during it, how overwhelming it can be if these matters are not continually looked at and dealt with along the way.

And now we come to the most difficult and involved question that has an effect on all the other matters we have discussed: How are we going to pay for everything we need during a health crisis?

Finances:

1. Do you have an accountant, financial planner, and/or advisor?

2. How much money do we have available?

3. What is our total income?

4. What resources do we have to generate income?

5. Are they jointly or individually owned?

6. What are your state's requirements for allowing you to get Medicaid?

7. My ill spouse is incapacitated. Can I sign her name to legal documents?

8. Where are all of your financial records?

9. Do you have a safety deposit box?

10. If you use a computer to keep financial records what is the program and what are the passwords?

11. Do you have a Durable Power of Attorney for all or partial financial decisions?

12. What is your IRS status?

13. Is there a Will or Trust Agreement, and where is it?

14. What are your investments and where are those records?

15. If you have a business, what plans have you made for its future without you?

16. Finally, in the event of your death, there are the many personal desires that need to be addressed such as:

    • Where do you wish to be buried, and have cemetery plots been purchased and other plans been made?

    • If cremation is desired, have those plans been made?

- What decisions have you made relative to distribution of valuables such as jewelry, furniture, and other items?
- Do you have any special desires for your burial service including, which I discovered during Anna's funeral process, Pall Bearers??

> "It is autumn; not without
> But within me is the cold.
> Youth and spring are all about:
> It is I that have grown old."

—Henry Wadsworth Longfellow, *Autumn Within*

There are obviously many other issues that will arise in individual cases, but if you only prepare for those listed herein you will be a long way ahead and able to smoothly handle whatever comes your way.

Nothing is more frustrating in going through this process than the road blocks put in your way by the very individuals who you are counting on to help you through the process.

The agents, administrators, key personnel, and customer service representatives—all of whom will one day face the same inquiries you are making—often act as if you are the cause of their difficulties rather than understanding that you are the customer, client, etc. And they are supposed to help you!

This not to defame the many wonderful persons who do know their role and reach out to make certain your need are taken care of.

Also, the long waits "On Hold" when calling various organizations takes its toll when time is of the essence.

Doing these tasks as part of your normal responsibilities early in your life, and then routinely updating them to fit your changing needs, as well as keeping all of your family and others involved in the process, will make your planning easy, smooth, and timely.

In closing this chapter, I want to be certain you understand that the questions pose above do not include the overwhelming medical questions which will need to be handled and which only those professionals you have confidence in can address.

From my own experience, as well as that of the many persons I spoke with over the past year, I would be cautious about running from doctor to doctor. Carefully select medical professionals in whom you have trust, and follow their advice and make your decisions based upon their recommendations.

———•———

A fifty-five-year-old man went to his doctor for his annual health check up. When the exam was over the man said to his doctor, "I am thinking about having a vasectomy. What do you think?"

Somewhat surprised, the doctor asked him, "Have you spoken to your family about this? After all, this is a major decision."

The man replied, "Yes, and they are in favor of it, sixteen to three."

SENIOR MOMENT #32

THE LOSS OF A LOVED ONE SHOULD CAUSE
A CELEBRATION OF THEIR LIFE

I've dreamed many dreams that never came true.
I've seen them vanish at dawn:
But I've realized enough of my dream, thank God,
To make me want to live on.

I've prayed many prayers when no answer came,
I've waited patient and long:
But answers have come to enough of my prayers
To make me keep praying on.

I've trusted many a friend who failed
And left me to weep alone:
But I've found enough of my friends true blue
To make me keep trusting on.

I've sown many seeds that fell by the way
For the birds to feed upon;
But I've held enough golden sheaves in my hand,
To make me keep sowing on.

I've drained the cup of disappointment and pain,
I've gone many days without song,
But I've sipped enough nectar from the rose of life
To make me want to live on.

—Anonymous

The earlier we engage with our loved ones, discuss the wonderful adventure life can be, and recognize that along the way we may find big boulders in our path which can only be removed using the strength of all of our loved ones and community, the happier our journey life will be.

Some have said to me, "Why do you repeat the words 'journey of life' so often in your book?" The answer is simply because that is what it is, and I have never met anyone who did not want their journey to be anything but fun.

From the very start of this book I have written about the aging process and what one needs to know and prepare for in order to live a full and complete life.

Yes, it was not always a smooth journey, and often we were frustrated and disappointed with the events as they unfolded, but remember that Edison had thousands of failures before he got it right, just once, and lit up the world.

Even though we think of death as the end of our presence bodily, if we have lived a meaningful life, helped others live theirs, and built a foundation of family and friendships, then the person may be gone, but our life's heritage lives on in the hearts and minds of those we have touched along the way.

Remember these poetic lines: "People die, but love lives on."

No matter how difficult it is to be a witness to the passing of a person we love and admire, I believe that we should not view that with sadness, but rather as a celebration of their life and the joy we had in having them in our lives.

What has saddened me the most in writing this book has been the number of persons near death who have told me that their biggest regret was not investing in time to develop friendships. As long as those you leave behind can feel your presence in their daily lives, your journey continues.

I thank you for staying with me during this journey and leave you with the words of one of the great women of the world, Mother Teresa:

"Life is an opportunity, benefit from it,
Life is beauty, admire it,
Life is a challenge, meet it,
Life is a duty, complete it,
Life is a game, play it,
Life is a promise, fulfill it,
Life is a sorrow, overcome it,
Life is a song, sing it,
Life is a struggle, accept it,
Life is a tragedy, confront it,
Life is an adventure, dare it,
Life is luck, make it,
Life is too precious, do not destroy it,
Life is life, fight for it."

From the start I have made it clear that one of the important elements of a happy life is humor. It seems to me that the following humorous story sums up the challenge that life presents. It comes to you through the kindness of a dear friend, Joan Vieweger, co-owner of the fine boutique Chocolate Firm Choclatique.

An elderly woman, Faye, is telling her friend Margaret that her doctor told he she needed to get some exercise. Faye said, "I twisted and turned, I bent down and stood up, I kneeled and waved my arms, and I jumped up and down. By the time I got the leotard on, the exercise class had ended."

Such is life, so enjoy every day.

At the start of this project I had three main objectives. To:

1. Honor the wonderful memories I had of my late wife, Anna.

2. Leave a legacy to my children, grandchildren, and great-grandchildren.

3. Share my own experiences as I moved through life to the eventual end.

What I did not expect to happen was that I would through the process get to really look at myself and discover who I really am and how the decisions I made along the way affected all of those around me, as well as how they affected me.

I have never been a person who lived his life backwards or with regrets. After all, what's done is done. What I can do is ensure that the next day in my life is better than the last one.

A close friend recently said to me that they understood how the loss of my wife and some very close friends, over the past year, must be a heavy burden for me to carry.

In fact, even though I miss them very much, I believe that while grieving for the loss of those great people who I loved and who have had a major impact on my life, it is important instead look at the positive affects those persons had on my life. This includes the way they, in real life, inspired me to be a better person and move on with living each day to make it better. Thus, keeping them, spiritually, a part of my growth.

I have become most comfortable with myself. I've realized that when I am gone others will judge me according to their experiences with our relationship and that the spirit of those I loved and lost in life, or through death, will always be with me and guide me through the days ahead.

As I close in on year eighty-five of my existence and I add up the negatives and positives of my life, I would like to share what I believe are the key things that have allowed me to prepare for death. These things, with some significant downsides, have helped me enjoy the trip. Perhaps by doing so it will inspire my readers to stop and carefully consider how these thoughts can help them get the most out of their journey:

- **Observe** and remember the way others you know and meet give you a positive feeling and incorporate that into your daily life.

- Learn to **forgive** those who offend you. It is certainly okay to be "temporarily" upset, but get over it. If the offense really so bad that you want nothing to do with the individual, that's okay. Separate them from your life, wish them well, and move on, but do not carry a grudge all the rest of your life.

- Do not **judge** others by what someone else tells you about them. Let your own experience guide you in relationships.

- Let go of **anger**. You only hurt yourself when you carry anger with you. Yes, we all get upset and sometimes want to scream and shout. However, remember that all issues play themselves out, and hanging onto the anger accomplishes nothing but raising your blood pressure and affecting your mood when interacting with others.

- No matter what the issue, remember that **good family relationships** at some point in your life are the most important of all relationships. Sooner or later they will be a major deterrent of how whether we live our lives out happily or not. We are in fact our "Brother's Keepers." I see this every day in working with the aged. Nothing is more clear proof of this than the reading of any Bible. Story after story, from century to century, the breakup and eventual reconciliation of family life is the basis for the happy ending of all biblical teachings.

- Understand the meaning of the word **love** and how to practice its various levels of applications. There is the love that exists between family members. We express love to our friends and acquaintances. Love of one's fellow workers shows your dedication to their success and to your own. There is also the tender love between two persons who are emotionally connected to each other. Finally, there is a special love that remains with us as a lifelong memory of those we have loved and lost—regardless of what role they played in our lives. How we express our love for others in each of the scenarios I have discussed is important to the growth of the relationship. Sometimes just expressing how you feel fits nicely. Sometimes, a warm embrace tells it all. At other times, when a friend is dealing with a tragedy of family death, the best expression of love is silence while being there as a demonstration of loving support. And in the case of romantic love, a combination of all of the above plus respecting your loved one's independence and looking at the future in the same direction, sends a clear message of what they mean to you.

- When I was a young man, my father taught me to never give up until I found the best in whatever I was doing or in my relationships. He taught me to **persevere** until I had. This lesson has served me well up until this very moment.

Life is challenging and frustrating, but if you live it right from the earliest days it can be exciting and rewarding. I still have my desires and goals and as I have discovered it is by persevering and persistence I have been able to achieve most of my dreams.

———◆———

"One friend said to another, 'Tell me, do you love me?'
The other replied, 'I love you deeply.'

The first friend asked, 'Do you know what gives me pain?'
The other responded, 'How can I know what gives you pain?'

"If you do not know what gives me pain," the friend replied,
"How can you say that you truly love me?"

—Morris Mandel

———◆———

It is most important, as we experience life and make decisions, to take into account both the words and actions of others whose paths we cross along the way.

How many times have we idolized leaders who preached goodness and character and discovered that while they spoke about high morality and good behavior, they themselves were discovered to be leading just the opposite kind of life?

At times in my own life I have had to stop and ask myself the same question, "Did I violate my own beliefs by taking this or that action? What right do I have to say one thing and do the opposite?"

What I have learned is that if I am unable to see what is painful to me, how can I see what is painful to those I love? These are the kinds of things that we need to talk about with our children when they are in their formative years and that we must, on a daily basis, consider with each action we take, each decision we make, and with each relationship we have.

No matter where my life has taken me, I am a happy man, for I have looked in the mirror, cried over my errors in judgment, applauded my good deeds, and communicated my feelings to all who I truly love and admire.

All of my deep-felt grief has been converted to the joy of having lived and known so many wonderful human beings.

I do not await death, although I know it will sometime arrive. I move on in life with this simple and easy to observe suggestion: Learn each day to help others, not because you have to or because it will make you look good, but because you want to and because it is right.

At the start of this book, I mentioned that I often quote others when I find something they have written or said that conveys my own feelings better than I can.

While the largest part of what you have read comes from deep within me, all of the quotations represent my personal thoughts, and every effort has been made to authenticate the source of the expressions which represent my beliefs.

And so as I come to the close of this writing I recall the words of an anonymous poet:

> Not, "How did he die?" But, "How did he live?"
> Not, "Where did he gain?" But, "What did he give?"
> These are the units to measure the worth
> Of a man as a man, regardless of birth.
>
> Not, "What was his station?" But had he a heart?
> And how did he play his God-given part?
> Was he ever ready with a word of good cheer
> To bring back a smile, to banish a tear?
>
> Not, "What was his shrine?" Nor, "What was his creed?"
> But had he befriended those really in need?
> Not, "What did the sketch in the newspaper say?"
> But how many were sorry when he passed away?

When you can look back over your life and say, "I did my best to meet these criteria," you can confidently say, "A job well done. I have traveled a happy road."

—◦—

Life's race well run
Life's work well done
Life's crown well won
Now comes rest

—◦—

Inscribed on the tomb of twentieth President James A. Garfield is the following Epitaph:

"It is essential that we enable young people to see themselves
as participants in one of the most exciting eras in history,
and to have a sense of purpose in relation to it."

—Nelson Rockefeller

In conclusion, let me share this thought with you: One of the most valuable assets you possess is awareness. When you wake up each day, if you cannot be happily aware of the beauty of the world you live in, the awareness of the opportunities that are yours to pursue—no matter what obstacles may be in your path—and the awareness of the wonderful relationships that await your participation, then no matter your age, you have already given up on life. Do not ever forget this as you travel life's road.

Checklist and More

If you have enjoyed this book and find my words of value, I encourage you to scan, print, and answer the questions included in this chapter for safekeeping:

For Home and Personal Issues:

- Do you have a list of all of your doctors and your relationship with them?
- Do you have a list of your insurance plans, how to contact them, and how they are paid for?
- Have you carefully gone through your home and evaluated it to be certain that the necessary safety conditions have been addressed?

- In case of a home maintenance problem (plumbing, electrical, gardening, heating, etc.) who are the vendors that provide you with those services?

- Do you have a home alert system in case you fall or need help, and how does it work?

- In case the help of a neighbor is needed, who are the ones you are close with and how do you reach them?

- Where in the home do you keep money, jewelry, and other valuables?

- Who is the insurer for those items mentioned above and how do you reach them?

- If you drive, where are the car keys kept, what insurance do you have, and how to we contact the insurer?

- Is the car paid for or leased, and who do you contact regarding those issues?

- What credit obligations do you have, how do you contact the creditors, and where are the credit cards and documentation connected to them?

- Who is going to be your primary caregiver and what authorization do they have to make decisions for you?

Insurance and Caregiver Questions:

- What kind of health, disability, long term, medication, and other health policies are you covered by?

- Do you have Medicare? Do you also have a supplemental health care policy that covers that portion of care that Medicare does not?

- Are your credit cards and other financial assets protected by credit defense programs?

- Do your policies cover home health care programs?

- Do you have list of contact information for all of the policies you have?

- In the case where you are the primary recipient of the benefits and other family members are covered under that policy, what happens to their benefits if you pass away?

- What are the waiting periods for activation of the pertinent policies?

- Are your doctors aware of who to call in case there is a danger to your health?

- What medications are you taking?

- Do all of your doctors know what other physicians are caring for your various health issues?

A Glossary and Some Definitions

Care Manager AKA Case Manager

A professional who is trained in how to plan, locate, and monitor appropriate social and medical services for individuals and their families who are not able to do so themselves. A well-trained Care Manager is invaluable in providing proper information. They advise on most issues involved in helping individuals and their families make the correct decisions in a timely manner.

Geriatric Care Manager

A Case or Care Manager who specializes in the assessment of an older adult's capabilities and can help in creating a care plan to address housing, medical, social, and other needs.

Geriatrician

A medical specialist who treats older persons. They are generally internal medicine or family practice physicians who have advanced training and certifications.

Caregiver

This is an individual who provides care to individuals who cannot care for themselves due to the various aging issues which have been described. This could be a friend, family member, or a paid individual. The care they give is generally in the area of personal needs such a dressing and bathing. It is important to keep in mind that such caregivers are usually not licensed.

Certified Nurse Aide (CNA)

A person who is trained and certified to provide general nursing care under the supervision of a registered nurse or therapist CAN's can help with all aspects of nursing care including help with bathing, eating and certain types of exercising.

Home Health Aide (HHA)

A professional who is trained to provide assistance with bathing, dressing, grooming, cooking and eating, as well as light housekeeping in order to help the patient live as independently as possible in a safe and friendly environment.

Home Health Agencies

A service (in the patient's home) that locates and manages health professionals who provide many of the services herein discussed. This includes but is not limited to: nursing, physical therapy, and/or personal care.

SENIOR MOMENT #33

THE TIME BETWEEN BIRTH AND DEATH SHOULD BE FILLED WITH JOY AND HAPPINESS—EVEN AS WE ENCOUNTER PAIN AND CHALLENGES ALONG THE WAY

It matters not how strait the gate,
How charged with punishment the scroll,
I am the master of my life,
I am the captain of my soul.

—William Ernest Henley

"Through Storms We Grow"

Rabbi Alexander Alan Steinbach

Life is meant to be lived joyfully and fully. Although there are bumps in the road, we must always be upbeat and understand that the bumps are there so that we know the difference.

In Rabbi Steinbach's book, from which the quote of this page comes, he raises some very interesting questions by asking, "What is the most precious thing a human being possesses?" He suggests that he obvious answer is "life."

He goes on to ask, "What kind of life does every individual crave?" He explains that he believes most persons would answer the question by saying, "a complete life."

And what are the ingredients of a complete life? Rabbi Steinbach suggests that there are four that derive from the biblical Abraham—Isaac story:

1. Music, poetry and the arts

2. Vision and lofty idealism

3. Culture and education

4. Hope

How wonderful and different our lives would be if parents, our educational system, mankind as a whole began at an early age to speak of the journey through life so that it ends we can each say, "I had a happy life."

Of all of these values, hope is the most important. Unless we are willing to accept that life and death are part of the process, we will never get the real joy that we can attain from life.

As a result of my personal experiences and research for this book, here are three things that are most obvious and should be wisely considered by you:

1. It is never too early to plan your life's journey.

2. It is never too late to live it.

3. Physical impairment is not an impediment to success.

The point of all of this is that no matter one's age, physical, or mental status, far too many talented, knowledgeable persons who still have much to give to society have given up on life and/or are being "stored" in their homes, institutions, or care centers waiting to die.

Yes, if we are not realistic about what we want to achieve in every stage of our life, we can fail, but if we plan carefully, make an honest effort, and retreat and revise our plan, then our chances of success are great.

We only fail when we stop trying. Age and illness may get in the way, but that should not stop us. I am in constant severe pain due to the operation I had on my leg in 2012 and there is no medicine that will relieve it, but I refuse to let that stop me from accomplishing my goals or living a happy life.

> At the final game of the World Series, a man takes a seat behind the home dugout. He sees that the seat next to him is empty and asks the person on the opposite side of the empty seat if someone is sitting there. He is told that the seat belongs to the man and that his wife was going to attend the game with him but that she had passed away. The man expresses his regrets the question of why the seat's

owner had not been able to find a friend or relative to attend the
game with him. The man replies, "They are all at the funeral."

It should be quite obvious when we look at the enormity of the issues involved in our
preparation for the end of our journey, as well as during it, how overwhelming it can be if
these matters are not continually looked at and dealt with along the way?

To my readers, life is too precious a gift to take for granted. The end of life is immensely
difficult for all involved.

Again, I can only hope I have made a small difference. Please use and add to these lists as
appropriate.

Thank you again.

I was sitting having breakfast with a friend when I heard music softly
playing and suddenly had this vision of two people dancing.

I quickly excused myself from the early morning feast and
went back to my apartment and wrote these words.

And saw the image of my beautiful bride who
was taken from me far too soon

I began to smile as I realized how fortunate we had
been to be for thirty years in each other's lives.

Memories of an Evening of Dance

The orchestra was playing a soft melody
And the lights in the room were romantically dim
I watched as he wrapped her in his arms so lovingly
And she placed hers gently around him.

They danced and they danced as if there were no end
And looked at each other with eyes filled with love
It was a sight to behold as a clear message it did send
That within each of us is tenderness implanted from Heaven above

As I stood there and watched them my eyes filled with tears

Remembering how Anna and I
Danced arm in arm all night long over the years
Never giving a thought to what was to come as time went by

We were filled with love and passion feeling as one
The joy of living a life so fulfilled
Wanting this dream we had with each other to go on an on
Gliding so gracefully around the room as the mu-
sic's warm rhythm in or hearts love did instill

As I slowly turned and walked out of that room
Wiping the tears from my eyes

A Special Message to My Readers

At the very beginning of this book I said that my purpose in writing it, in addition to being a tribute to my beloved Anna, was to recognize that the one certain thing that was going to happen to all of us after birth was that we are going to die. I explained that we need to prepare for that by living our lives in such a way that when the end comes, we can truly say I lived, I loved, and I enjoyed the wonderful journey that I took.

Throughout the book I have shared stories with you about individuals that I've met over the years, was associated with during their journey of life, and how they brought happiness to themselves and others despite aging problems.

Before we could publish this book, several of those individual passed on. In acknowledging that, I also can say with all sincerity that they enjoy their life until the very end. We too should we dedicate ourselves to the goal of being able to leave this world all the better because we were in it.

Until we meet again, I leave you with the following heartfelt message: May you live your life every day sharing your love with those you know. I hope you enjoy your life in the same beautiful way that is described in my poem.

The Flourishing Rose Bush

When I was a sixteen-year-old kid and saw an eighty-five year old man
Holding hands with a beautiful woman slightly young-
er than him, I asked myself, "How is that possible?"

But now that I am that eighty-five-year-old, sixteen-year-old kid
I think I finally know the answer

Love is like the seed of a rose bush
When you plant it in the Garden of Eden

And then you feed and nourish it
Letting the sun and the moon shine upon it

You soon smell the rich aroma and feel the love
That comes from Heaven above

Credits

This book is a work of art produced by Incorgnito Publishing Press.

Taylor A. Basilio
Editor

Janice Bini,
Chief Reader

Stephen Gonzaga
Artist

Daria Lacy
Designer

Michael Conant
Publisher

May 2015
Incorgnito Publishing Press
mconant@incorgnitobooks.com